Women and Substance Use

Women and Substance Use

Elizabeth Ettorre

Rutgers University Press
New Brunswick, New Jersey

First published in cloth and paperback in the United States of America by
Rutgers University Press, 1992

First published in cloth and paperback in the United Kingdom by
The Macmillan Press Ltd

Library of Congress Cataloging-in-Publication Data
Ettorre, E. M.
Women and substance use / Elizabeth Ettorre.
p.   cm.
Includes bibliographical references and index.
ISBN 0-8135-1863-6 (cloth) — ISBN 0-8135-1864-4 (pbk.)
1. Women—Substance use.   2. Feminist theory.   I. Title.
RC546.5.W65E77   1992
362.29'082—dc20   92-7113
                                                    CIP

Printed in Hong Kong

To mother, whose energy, warmth and humour spark my creativity

Contents

Acknowledgements

This book is the result of my experiences as a woman research sociologist in the field of substance use.

Jo Campling, my editor with endless patience, invited me to do this book. She deserves a special vote of thanks.

There are a number of friends and colleagues who have encouraged me to write this book. They include Susanne MacGregor and all my colleagues at Birkbeck College, Mary Treacy, Jan Holland, Geoff Hunt, Jan Waterson, Maureen Sears, Martin Eede and Michael Bryant.

John Whitton at ISDD library provided me with endless cups of tea and lovely smiles of encouragement. Nick Dorn (ISDD) very kindly sat down with me and gave me many helpful suggestions for a title for this book. He and his colleague, Nigel South have consistently supported my work on women.

I should like to thank all my FINRRAGE colleagues, including Patricia Spallone, Debbie Steinberg, Marilyn Cranshaw, Penny Bainbridge, Sarah Franklin, Noe Mendelle and Annette Burfoot, who have given me enormous support.

Very special thanks go to my Finnish colleagues, Pia, Toffy, Sami and Maaria at the Nordic Council for Alcohol and Drugs Research (NAD). I spent two months at NAD in 1991 (April to June) as a visiting researcher in Helsinki, Finland. I believe their warmth, kindness and generosity provided a creative environment in which I was able to complete this text. Also I should like to thank Professor Elianne Riska, Director of the Institute of Women's Studies, Åbo Akademi University, Turku, Finland, for her helpful comments on Chapter 3.

Over the years, two women in particular have provided me with inspiration because of their commitment to the needs of women:

Professor Hilary Rose (University of Bradford) and Dr Dorothy Black (formerly of the Department of Health). I am very grateful to them both and appreciate their faith in me.

Finally I am most grateful to all the women users who have spoken to me about their experiences. I hope they will find this book challenging and worthwhile.

ELIZABETH ETTORRE

Note: The author and publishers wish to thank Basil Blackwell Publishers Ltd for permission to reproduce an extract from *Tabacco* by F. P. Wilson. Every effort has been made to contact all the copyright-holders, but if any have been inadvertently omitted the publishers will be pleased to make the necessary arrangement at the earliest opportunity.

Introduction: discovering a 'non-field'

Dis-covering: uncovering the Elemental Reality hidden by the hucksters, frauds, and framers of phallocracy; finding the treasures of women's Memory, Knowledge, History that have been buried by the grave diggers of patriarchal re-search . . . (Mary Daly in cahoots with Jane Caputi, *The Wickedary*)

Uncovering women substance users

As a woman researcher who has worked in the 'addiction' field for the past 15 years, I have seen consistently a need to offer a clear account of women and substance use written 'by a woman for women'. The desire to write this account grew as I found many of my colleagues, whether researchers or clinicians, women or men, to be resistant to a women-oriented perspective in the area.

With this level of resistance, two very basic principles need to be injected into this field if a women-oriented perspective is to develop: (1) that we need to be somewhat familiar with the social scientific way of viewing the world and, in particular, with the way in which the notion of gender has had an impact on recent developments in the social sciences; and (2) that we are open both theoretically and methodologically to an approach which is sensitive to the needs of women as a social group. Until these principles are accepted it is difficult to assume that addiction studies will allow the creation of a much needed environment in which the production of feminist knowledge is a real possibility.

Within 'addiction studies', feminist ideas are viewed as unconventional, if not antagonistic to traditional ideas held by 'addiction' professionals. 'Addiction professionals' have the power not only to define what 'substance-abusing women' represent (that is, diseased, polluted and/or bad women) but also to establish the boundaries for debate, making the needs of women invisible. In reality, women who experience problems with a whole variety of substances are usually left feeling stigmatised, marginalised and demoralised.

In writing this book I believe it is important to 'set the record straight' for women. Therefore the main aim of this text is to offer a feminist analysis in the field of substance use, a field of thought dominated traditionally by members of the medical profession who tend to be male, white and middle-class. I would suggest further that if, in this field, as in other fields of research, gender was recognised as a key concept, a major breakthrough would occur: the women's issue would no longer be viewed with distaste, if not intense discomfort by these 'phallocrats' (the male professionals defining the issue).

The difficulties of introducing critical work on gender as a valid area of research in this field must not be underestimated. Until recently the images, situations and needs of women substance users were largely unacknowledged, both within the treatment and within the research world and this area of research has been referred to as a 'non-field' (Kalant, 1980). As Blume (1990a) suggests, health professionals have been continually guided by the stereotype of the fallen woman.

Most work written about women substance users focuses, with few exceptions, on those seeking help or treatment. Analyses therefore need to be offered with reference to women substance users who are not drawn from 'clinical populations'. A theoretical approach should be offered which establishes a balance between individualistic, processual (that is, symbolic interactionist, pyschologistic) explanations and structural explanations (those sensitive to the overall social issues of class, gender and race). My contention is that, thus far, explanations about women offered in this area remain generally uncritical and ahistorical. Furthermore it would be futile for the reader to consider that major lines of feminist critique in the addiction field can be outlined in this text. This is because a feminist critique on substance misuse does not exist. Few, if any feminist scholars have written about women and addictions.

Given the above, the reader needs to be guided through the key strands of thought which this text, based on a feminist account, attempts to explore. In other words, if the field of women and addiction has been a 'non-field', what are the repercussions theoretically and practically on both a national and an international scale? While making this exploration, the reader needs to become aware of some of the historical reasons why the field has been resistant to the notion of gender as well as to an approach sensitive to the needs of women. The reader needs to know some of the reasons why the development of a gender-sensitive perspective on addictions remains in an 'infancy stage' of development.

The traditional perspective

To emphasise what has been stated previously the field of substance use has been dominated both in theoretical orientation and in clinical practice by members of the medical profession. Specifically psychiatrists, as proponents of the 'disease model of addiction', have been influential in determining how the 'disease' of addiction should be treated. With special reference to alcoholism, Jellinek (1960, pp. 35–51), contended that it is a type of 'disease entity'. The 'species of alcoholism' should be considered as 'disease processes or symptoms of disease processes'. In effect the species of alcoholism 'can breed'.

Proponents of the disease model of addiction have prioritised research questions such as: how does this disease spread?; what are the patterns and extent of the non-medical/medical use of drugs?; and what is the prevalence and incidence of various types of addiction?.

While the study of addiction is framed by these sorts of 'scientific' questions, 'expert' investigators, such as epidemiologists, are called upon to find the answers, perceived as the 'truth'. Epidemiology is defined literally as the 'study of or science of epidemics'. A more formal definition of epidemiology, offered by the World Health Organisation, is 'the study of the distribution of diseases or conditions in a population and of factors that influence that distribution' (quoted in Edwards, 1978). While it is important to look at the patterns of 'diseases' on a worldwide scale, this sort of emphasis, in my view, has taken concern away from more important questions such as: what are the real politics involved in both the illegal and legal drug trade?; why, in recent years, has the third world become the dumping ground for unwanted cigarettes, alcohol and pharmaceuticals produced in wealthy industrialised nations?; what is the relationship between social inequality and substance use and why is this latter issue consistently ignored? On a more subtle level, traditional perspectives in the field have also been powerful in designating the 'stereotypical' images which pertain to both men and women. While these images differ for both sexes, images of women, whether as substance users themselves or as partners of male users, distort the reality of women's lives.

While in recent years there has been increased talk of the excess in number of male substance users over female substance users or, simply, the 'male preponderance' in the literature and treatment world, this imbalance is usually justified by evoking 'outdated' social myths and attitudes. For example, one author, concerned that men more than women appear to experiment with drugs or to be noticed by treatment agencies because of their drug use, illustrates the above point very clearly:

> There may be many reasons for the greater likelihood of males to use drugs non-medically. There could be biological or personality differences between the sexes which predispose males more than females to indulge in drug use. Males are more aggressive . . . There is evidence that hostility is a trait associated with drug dependence, so perhaps females are generally psychologically less disposed than males to become drug dependent . . . (Plant, 1981, p. 258)

In the event that some women do get involved with drugs, they are seen to have a greater problem and to be more deviant or more psychologically disturbed than their male counterparts. This implies that the consciousness of those making these erroneous assumptions needs to be raised before women substance users gain equal treatment, whether institutional or not, in relation to men.

On the other hand, if women are seen in partnerships with men who use substances, they are seen as 'etiological agents' (that is, helping to cause the addiction) or 'complicating the illness' (Jackson, 1962). In a classic British study on alcoholism, two psychiatrists refer to the wife of an alcoholic as 'a determining or at least an aggravating factor' (Kessel and Walton, 1965, p. 108). The idea that women victims of assault after a heavy bout of drinking may be in someway responsible for male violence is subtly suggested in today's literature (Shepherd, Irish, Scully and Leslie, 1989). That women are seen as colluding with 'their men' or as 'active victims' has, in my view, had subtle effects in the area of domestic violence. The implication is that, while the link between substance use, particularly alcohol, and domestic violence has remained hidden, if not subverted, women, as recipients of this violence, have been viewed as in some way responsible for it.

In this context allow me to share with the reader a fascinating as well as disturbing anecdote. While carrying out a national study of Alcohol Treatment Units (ATUs) in England and Wales (Ettorre 1984, 1985a, 1985b, 1985c), the author conducted an interview with a consultant psychiatrist who, at that time, ran an ATU on the grounds of a large psychiatric hospital. The author, then research sociologist, enquired about the kinds of people who had become patients and had been finally admitted to his ATU for treatment. The psychiatrist replied enthusiastically, emphasising the need for his staff to maintain a peaceful or, to be more precise, a 'non-disruptive treatment environment'. His response was most illuminating. He said: 'We don't take any violent people. Of course, if a man beats his wife, we don't count that as violence.' Need one say more than that women are damned if they drink and damned if their husbands drink?

Developing a feminist framework

In writing this book on women and substance use, the author feels the need to distance herself from the majority of her 'addiction' colleagues and to argue for a critical approach which views substance use as a complex social issue with specific political implications rather than as an epidemiological concern (that is, as an individual disease, a psychiatric disorder or even an implicit moral failing). Simply, a basic contention of this book is that there is a need for a theoretical perspective, highlighting social divisions in society and focusing on the variety of historical, cultural and political forces which shape the entire substance use issue.

Linked with this contention is the demand to recognise key issues which need to be unearthed if workers are to share a collective view, responsive to the needs of women substance users. To present a broad overview mindful of women's experience, is an overwhelming task, viewed with dismay by colleagues who are insensitive to the needs of women or afraid of feminist ideas. Nevertheless the author's search, directed by her experience as a woman as well as her observations as a feminist researcher, has been worthwhile and should cast a critical light on traditional frameworks in the field.

Viewed purely as consumer products, both legal and illegal addictive substances are beneficial to prevailing economic structures, dependent on the multinational alcohol industry (Cavanagh and Clairmonte, 1985), the global heroin market (Lewis, 1985), the growth of the pharmaceutical industry (Ettorre, 1985d), the exploitation of new drug markets, such as cocaine and cannabis (Sargent, 1983; Henman, 1985; Maylon, 1985) and in Britain the £50 million a day gained by the Chancellor from tobacco sales (Edwards, 1984). It is fair to say that most research in the addiction field ignores these important structural issues. Also it has already been demonstrated that, particularly in the alcohol field, little attention is paid to global, political and economic forces (Singer, 1986).

On the one hand, addictive substances are rooted in the very fabric of our society. On the other hand, the use of these substances runs 'counter to the ethos of a disciplinary society' (Smart, 1984, p. 34). Furthermore correlations between unemployment and addiction are played down, whilst drug scares or what Kohn (1987) refers to as 'Narcomania' are used to divert attention away from other more important social issues. What we need to understand in the addiction field is that 'legal and illegal are political and often arbitrary categorizations; use and abuse are medical or clinical distinctions' (Hoffman, 1987).

Let us look briefly at the usefulness of the concept of substance use as a notion which helps to broaden the somewhat narrow confines of traditional debates within addiction studies. In this discussion we will also look at some earlier conceptions and images of 'addiction' that still exist today.

The 'hierarchy' of drugs

While the majority if not all of the discussions in the field of addiction focus on substances which are 'mind-altering' or 'psychotropic', the discussions presented in this book will consider as relevant *any* substance, chemical or otherwise, that alters mood, perception or consciousness *and/or* is seen to be misused to the apparent detriment of society and the individual. By replacing 'drug use' with the notion of 'substance use' we are explicitly including new discourses on bodily management and regulation within our frame of reference. The terms 'heroin misuse', 'tranquilliser addiction' and 'alcohol abuse' are all useful in denoting particular biochemical and physiological processes. However, from the viewpoint of women, 'substance use' is a more illuminating notion. (This will be discussed in more detail in the following chapter.)

Given the above, one could argue rightly that traditional discussions in the field of addiction should be extended to include a consideration of those substances which are not intrinsically 'mind-altering', but which cause any number of problems for an individual. Specifically, with reference to current debates within the addiction field, there is a need to demonstrate how the term 'substance use/abuse' rather than 'drug use/abuse' or 'addiction' is more relevant to women's everyday lives. Establishing links with women's oppression, a growing body of feminist literature looks at the consequences of women's use and abuse of substances, such as food, as a type of addictive substance (Orbach, 1978, 1986; Chernin, 1981; Lawrence, 1987).

The notion of substance use suggests that feminist literature in the area of eating and food could have a significant place within the traditional discourse on addiction. Simply, the notion is perhaps more sensitive to the gender issue than terms such as addiction, drug misuse or substance misuse. For example, anorexia nervosa exists as a diagnostic category for both men and women, yet the terms anorexics and boulimics, tend to conjure up images of emaciated females (Orbach, 1986) rather than emaciated males. Additionally the term anorexia nervosa as a diagnostic label 'has become increasingly popular among medical professionals, suggesting an increased prevalence of the illness' (Turner, 1987, p. 106) and a further singling out of women.

While helping to expand the context of traditional debates, the notion of substance use allows us to recognise more easily what I would call 'the hierarchy of drugs'. For example, within society the use of drugs involves a socially constructed hierarchy ranging from 'good' drugs at the top of the hierarchy to 'bad' drugs at the bottom. It is quite common within a drug-using society for most, if not all individuals to be dependent upon a variety of consumer products. These include tea, coffee, cigarettes, sweets and, as we have already seen above, food itself. These consumer products or commodities, whether they contain substances such as caffeine, nicotine or glucose, are seen to be good or at least socially acceptable if individuals become addicted to them. These 'addictive' substances remain at the top of the hierarchy of drugs. Alcohol, a licit psychotropic drug, is viewed as a substance which, if used in moderation, enhances social gatherings. In this way it too is placed towards the top of the hierarchy of drugs. On the other hand, illicit drugs, such as opiates, cannabis or cocaine or any drugs obtained illegally are socially condemned and their use may lead to imprisonment if not some form of social containment. As these drugs are at the bottom of the hierarchy of drugs, users of these drugs experience social exclusion from the dominant culture. They are 'marginalised, stigmatised and outcasts' (MacGregor, 1986). They are seen to have chaotic life styles. From a different standpoint, tranquillisers which, if used on a long-term basis, have adverse effects on the majority of users. They are seen for women as 'good' or socially necessary to maintain domestic bliss or the stability of the family (Ettorre, 1985d). They tend to be placed high on the hierarchy of drugs.

Implicit in this hierarchy is the view not only that some substances are better than others but also that some substances are more polluting both chemically *and* socially than others. In a paper entitled 'Internal Pollution' (subtitled 'Poisoned People'), Warburton (1978) defines internal pollution as the 'state when the purity of the internal environment of our bodies is destroyed'. He points out that the notion of internal pollution has received scant attention in the field of substance use. He also argues that it is easy for those with an awareness of drugs in society to blame over-prescribing doctors; to criticise the marketing strategies of the pharmaceutical or the alcohol industry and to see the failure of governments to curb, if not control, the illegal global trade in heroin. However, for Warburton, the consumers of drugs are to be blamed. These substance 'abusers' whose bodies become the internal environments for pollution actually collude in this pollution process by demanding drugs. Significantly Warburton makes a moral judgement: substance abusers pollute themselves as well as their social environments.

I would argue that this is a clear case of victim blaming which gives us faint reflections of an earlier nineteenth-century 'public health' concern with social contagion. As one author tells us:

> Public health as opposed to individual sickness was a newly emergent concept premised upon an understanding of society as an organic whole which could become sick in its entirety. But public health was not identified as solely at risk from physiological disease, but also from behaviours defined as socially problematic . . . The practice of drug taking began to be re-interpreted as a threat to the new concept of public health. (Smart, 1984)

Substance use as a threat to public health

Substance use destroys the purity of the social environment or social hygiene which, in the nineteenth century, demanded temperance, proper diet and sanitation amongst the working class as the middle class sought to protect themselves from disease. While at that time drug use was not seen as a contagious disease, it was viewed as a physical disease and a 'scientifically identified threat to society' (Smart, 1984). In turn the 'addict' was 'singled out as a distinct, abnormal personality' (Berridge, 1988) as well as being separated out as a specific type of person whom 'only the medical profession was competent to treat' (Berridge and Edwards, 1981, p. 170).

Alongside these public health notions was the trend towards the scientific analysis of diet, the outcome of debates around issues to do with urban poverty, efficiency and the management of prisons and asylums. While food consumption became the measure for poverty in the ninteenth century, drug consumption becomes the measure of the growth of the ideologies of despair amongst working-class youth today. As one anthropologist (Burr, 1985) suggests: 'Drugs became another example of the way individuals and young people in particular use the body as a medium of expression for solving their problems'.

However, for women, using their bodies as a medium of expression for solving their problems has particular implications. Objectively the female body 'has been mankind's most popular subject for adoration and myth and also for judgement, ridicule, aesthetic adoration and violent abuse' (Brownmiller, 1984, p. 12). If women are seen to 'abuse' in any way their already abused bodies, they are seen to be worse than their male counterparts. This is because these women are seen to defile and indeed to desecrate the sacred symbol of their sexual essence: their bodies which house their wombs or reproductive power. While the female body is the embodiment of women's reproductive nature, substance abuse is seen as an attack on women's nature. A substance-abusing woman is the quintessence of a wicked woman defiling her body with harmful substances. Let us now turn our attention to the contents of this book.

The structure of this book

As suggested in the above discussions, this text will focus on a variety of substances (whether or not they are mind-altering). We will look specifically at women's use of alcohol, prescribed drugs (specifically minor tranquillisers), heroin, tobacco and food. Given this focus, there is a need for future work on women's use of solvents, cannabis, cocaine, OTCs (over the counter drugs), steroids, major tranquillisers, hallucinogens and coffee: all substances omitted in the text. Using the term 'substance use' throughout, the text is a direct challenge to ideas regarding women in the addiction field. More significantly, it is a deliberate attempt to put forward a feminist perspective as well as a women-oriented response which is rooted in the identity and consciousness of women substance users.

The reader should be aware that this is not a text-book in the traditional sense. For each of the topics an attempt is made to discuss existing material, to outline the current state of play and to offer a critique from a feminist point of view. However, as the reader will quickly sense, the feminist critique is paramount for each chapter and the discussions of existing research and literature are not uniform. This is because there is more material on women for some topics than others and factual statistical information on women substance users is patchy. For example, the reader will be aware that there is more information presented in the chapters on alcohol and smoking than in the chapters on food dependence and heroin. This reflects the general state of play within the respective fields.

Additionally, because men more often than women are viewed as the real substance abusers, there tends to be more information available on these male consumers in each of the specified areas. This fact makes it extremely difficult to develop a sense of comprehensiveness on women while male clinicians, researchers and consumers remain dominant in the field. Developing an understanding of women in each of the chosen fields is therefore more difficult than one might expect. By making a women-oriented perspective paramount, this text attempts to redress this imbalance. Each chapter is prefaced by a quotation taken from the work of a woman writer. This strategy aims to focus the reader's attention consistently on the awareness that the text is women-oriented. Let us now look briefly at the structure and the content of the following chapters.

Chapter 1 outlines in some detail the need for a women-oriented perspective on women and substance use and sets the text firmly within a feminist perspective. Four interrelated issues will be discussed: substance use as a 'gender-illuminating issue'; the 'unacceptable' and 'acceptable' faces of dependency; the development of a women-oriented methodology in the field of substance use; and whether substance use and pleasure is relevant for women. It is argued that, given the major theoretical and methodological drawbacks in the field of addiction studies, we need an approach which is sensitive to the needs of women as a social group. We are left with a clear picture of how masculinist ways of thinking can be challenged effectively in the substance use field.

Chapters 2, 3, 4, 5 and 6 have similar formats, providing insights into the literature and work emerging from both clinicians' and researchers' concentration on specific substances, including food. In the introduction to each chapter the author will identify the 'key issues' which are a necessary part of a critical framework in the development of a women-oriented perspective. Then the following discussions weave these key issues together as each chapter progresses. It is hoped that the reader, whether a student or a teacher, a researcher or a clinician, male or female will develop their own insights as they read the text. All five chapters will be based on the underlying assumption that there is a great need for a clear feminist perspective in the field of substance use. Also an overall theme running throughout these chapters is the idea that regardless of the widespread feminist concern with the notion of dependency, different substances used and 'abused' by women warrant separate analyses. Distinct analyses will help to expose one of the major misconceptions put forward by both clinicians and researchers in the field: women substance users are a homogeneous group. Consistently this major conception will be challenged.

In Chapter 2 special emphasis will be placed on the way women problem drinkers challenge traditional female stereotypes and roles related to the identity of a 'real woman'. Notions such as 'polyproblems', the double standard and the 'alcohol dependence syndrome' *vis-à-vis* alcohol-dependent women will be examined. A critical examination of the foetal alcohol syndrome will be presented. While challenging traditional concepts in the field, we will begin to see the level of resistance to a women-centred perspective. Women's social agency is seen as necessary in order to confront the unsympathetic tactics used with regard to women in this area.

Chapter 3 will focus on the woman 'minor' tranquilliser user, emerging from the 'private' sphere and, perhaps, posing less of a threat to the established order than her heroin- or alcohol-using counterparts. As both 'strung-out patient' and 'dutiful wife', she is managed and manageable in an environment legitimated by male authority: that of her husband and her doctor. Tranquilliser use may be a woman's/housewife's only recourse to comfort and relief from stress. Regardless of the initial reason or reasons for a woman actively consuming benzodiazepines, she perpetuates the image of women as 'passive consumers'. This chapter will discuss in detail other areas of concern *vis-à-vis* women tranquilliser users: the health care industry, the medical profession and the pharmaceutical industry. A major strand of thought in this chapter is that, unless society changes at deep levels, women have no remedy for their forced alienation from themselves or for their inferiority.

In Chapter 4 we will focus primarily on heroin, an illegal drug. It has been suggested in the field that women heroin users in the public sphere represent femininity 'misplaced', 'defied' and 'defiled' (Perry, 1979). Specifically the female 'junkie' and/or 'pusher' is the embodiment of a woman who rejects her femininity. In reality she is a 'non-woman' in the public sphere and her visibility is a direct challenge to the established, patriarchal order. Key discussions presented in this chapter include: how heroin can be seen as a masculine drug; why women who use heroin are perceived as polluted women and as having spoiled their identity; women's experience of the drug treatment system; and women in relation to injecting drug use, prostitution and AIDS.

Similarities between the targeting strategies of the tobacco industry and the alcohol industry will be made in Chapter 5. After examining women's increased consumption of tobacco in recent years, we will look at a series of feminist notions such as women's praxis, caring, pleasure and 'patriarchal pain' in order to build a framework of understanding in this area of substance use. We will also look at symbols of smoking in the public and private spheres, smoking and poverty and smoking and ethnicity. It is hoped that challenges to existing work in this area will be made and that the reader will see the women and smoking issue in a new light.

Chapter 6 focuses on the sensitive area of women's dependence on food. Discussions will attempt to incorporate feminist concerns, emerging both in Britain and the United States . On the one hand, some feminists, such as Orbach (1978) have argued that 'fat is a feminist issue' and that women must look critically at their reasons for overeating. On the other hand, feminists similar to Schoenfielder and Wieser (1983) argue that being fat is OK and that one should actively work for the liberation of fat women who ultimately reject the imposed images of an acceptable woman in a male-oriented society. This chapter explores this contradiction and focuses on a number of key issues, including the politics of global food consumption; the politicisation of women's bodies; food addiction as substance misuse; images of the ideal female body; women's flesh and women's bodies and a feminist view of the politics of dieting. We conclude that all women need to be women of substance.

The remaining two chapters systematise the text's feminist and women-oriented perspective from both a practical and a theoretical standpoint. Within the context of the women's health movement, Chapter 7 looks at recent developments in the feminist response to substance use. Areas for exploration include discussions on the issues of 'process addiction'; the women's health movement; the development of a feminist epistemology and the difference between the clinical and structural models of self-help. Special reference will be made to the types of feminist strategies which should be used within the substance use field in order to mobilise women in this area. The increasing visibility of these strategies needs some consideration if changes are to occur.

The concluding chapter attempts to identify the common themes and notions which have emerged throughout the text and to draw them together. These themes and notions include the quest for pleasure; autonomy and empowerment; the link between sex and drugs; Physical Ultimacy and physical intimacy; decreasing pain; coming to terms with one's body; and addicting forces and women.

It will become clear that, regardless of the substance used or 'abused', women need to build an alternative creative response challenging the pervasive dogmatism which exists in the substance use field. By this stage of the text, the reader should be aware that this field remains impotent and insensitive to the needs of women. A feminist approach is urgently needed and this book is a modest attempt to generate interest in this type of approach, so that women substance users, as well as those researchers and clinicians sympathetic to a women-sensitive response, will be more able than before to put forward women-oriented ideas and to work together towards the establishment of a collective, feminist view.

1

Moving beyond 'masculinist' truths

> Women's early centrality and solidity was
> essentially familial, a connection of mother
> with daughters and granddaughters, sisters
> with each other and with nieces and grand-
> nieces, and among cousins. Breaking this core
> is essential to asserting male superiority or
> supremacy. (Marilyn French, *Beyond Power:
> on Women, Men and Morals*)

Introduction

As suggested in the introduction, the field of addiction studies has
been resistant both theoretically and methodologically to an
approach which is sensitive to the needs of women as a social
group. As in other fields of social research, there is a need for a
sound theoretical framework challenging methodologies which
'ignore sexual divisions and do not "see" the experiences of
women' (Roberts, 1981, p. 15). Simply, there is a need for
approaches on substance use highlighting the social construction
of gender. While this chapter mirrors what Spender (1981, p. 199)
would refer to as a 'feminist venture into male territory', it begins to
explore the ways in which the experience of women substance users
can be recognised and valued.

The first step of this venture is to begin creating a critical framework in which the production of feminist knowledge becomes a real possibility within this field. This chapter attempts to outline key issues which place the women and substance use issue within a feminist perspective. Given that there are problems, conflicts and difficulties in defining women's relationship to substance use as a feminist issue, a discussion of how we can overcome these obstacles is timely.

To gain a clear view on any social issue related to women is to uncover a unique sense of history or 'herstory', to be more precise, fraught with struggle and pain as well as charged with human dignity and worth. While a clear view on women and substance use does not escape this unique sense of 'herstory', it does make visible powerful images specific to our substance-abusing cultures. These images of women should be explored within an integrative and empowering framework. In other words, we need images of women substance users that empower rather than stigmatise or victimise them. We also need to learn how to recognise these images while we are creating an alternative framework sensitive to the needs of women. In effect we are attempting to look at a well-established area of study in a different light. It is hoped that the perspective put forward will clarify issues for further debate.

Four interrelated issues will be discussed: substance use as a 'gender-illuminating issue'; the 'unacceptable' and 'acceptable' faces of dependency; the development of a women-oriented methodology in the field of substance use; and whether substance use and pleasure is relevant for women. It is hoped that the reader will gain a distinct view of the way 'masculinist' ways of thinking can be appropriately challenged in the substance use field.

The need for a feminist perspective which moves beyond masculinist 'truths'

Objectively we live in stress-filled societies in which women's social position and the nature of the female role is more conducive to mental illness than psychological well-being (Brown and Harris, 1978; Chesler, 1972; Walker, 1984; Penfold and Walker, 1984); women are viewed as major health care consumers (Graham, 1984; Doyal, 1981); dependence on substances, addictive or otherwise, is a potentially important factor in any woman's life (DAWN, 1984; 1985a; 1985b; 1986); and, furthermore, the general concept, dependency, has a different meaning for men and women (Graham, 1983).

Within the field of addiction, these issues remain hidden and, ultimately, are not recognised as important. Given this fact, it is not surprising that addiction research disregards the gender order with its established social division of patriarchy. As a result the significance of substance use for women as a social group is concealed, if not actively subverted and hidden.

By centring on men, the most socially 'visible' participants within our drug-using cultures, 'scientific' research in the addiction field tends to uphold traditional, patriarchal images of men and women. As a result a distorted view of women is presented. The development of a feminist analysis, similar to the critique offered within the area of science and technology, would be useful in order to give us a more balanced picture of women. Only then could we begin to move effectively beyond what Rose (1986) calls 'masculinist realities' and challenge patriarchal notions oppressive to women.

Within the field of addiction, the centrality of these notions (that men are socially dominant and active participants in the drug-using culture and women are socially subordinate and relatively passive participants) has meant that the situations and needs of women were largely unacknowledged and unrecognised within both the treatment and the research world. Also it has been shown how experts in the general mental health field produce 'gender-laden rhetoric' in their diagnostic practice (Holstein, 1987). It could be suggested further that gender-laden rhetoric is also rampant in the addiction field.

Traditionally the lack of a body of knowledge about women and substance use led those, specifically psychiatrists and clinical psychologists working in the field, to assume that substance use was primarily a 'man's disease' or a 'male problem'. Women were effectively ignored and excluded from these analyses. We see this very clearly in the alcohol field. When explanations of normal social drinking were provided, these were based on assumptions such as 'developing a taste for drink, a palate, is a male attribute'; 'real men drink real ale' or 'within our drug using culture men learn to drink, while women do not' (Gofton, 1983). These sorts of false assumptions do not in any way challenge the partiality to men prevalent in the alcoholism field, nor do they help to question the belief that alcoholism is predominantly a male problem.

While there have been attempts, particularly by feminist researchers or those sympathetic to a feminist approach, to include women firmly within the addiction field (Ahlstrom, 1983; Suurla, 1989), male bias (Vanicelli and Nash, 1984) and the sexist assumption that women are no different from their male counterparts (Richmond, 1981) appear to remain as operating principles in the field.

It is interesting to point out that it is only in recent years that any links between alcohol and domestic violence or violence against women have been made (Kaufman Kantor and Straus, 1987; Morgan, 1981; Room, 1980) and there is a general lack of interest in examining the established, masculinist drinking traditions as a form of social control. In this context, Hunt and Saterlee's (1987) work is an exceptional investigation, exposing the culture of female drinking as a separate activity, if not a challenge to this masculinist tradition. That gender arrangements are taken seriously in this anthropological study of pub culture is a welcomed change, as well as a necessary step towards the establishment of a feminist perspective in the area.

The author has already outlined elsewhere (Ettorre, 1986a), with special reference to alcohol sociology, strategies helpful for the establishment of this perspective. However it should be emphasised here that this is a unique process. It involves a new way of seeing and the transformation of traditional views into what we could call 'gender-illuminating notions'. These notions appropriately reflect the somewhat mundane and invisible realities of women's everyday lives. We need these notions because without them women substance users remain isolated and excluded from proper understanding and treatment.

Substance use as a 'gender illuminating notion'

To gain a full insight into any women's issue, such as women and substance use, we need to be aware that there are many complex issues that are not visible at first glance. We need to unearth the genealogy of women's collective survival in relation to 'addictive' substances. Simply, we need to discover a particular 'herstory' that reflects the constant struggle for women to maintain their female integrity and self-worth in a substance-abusing, stress-filled society. That this society is dependent economically, politically and culturally on a 'cushioning process', provided by a variety of chemical comforts, shows the extent to which addiction and indeed stress have become 'normal', established facts of life. As Gossop (1982) shows, the irony associated with this sort of cultural process is that chemical comforts can provide only temporary relief. None of them solves the 'normal' problems of living and, for women, the notion of 'problems of living' has specific social and cultural ramifications.

In this context women researchers in the field have looked at the consequences of 'a tranquilliser trap for women' (Melville, 1984); 'women bottling it up' (Curran and Golombok, 1985); 'cigarettes as ladykillers' (Jacobson, 1981); 'women under the influence' (McConville, 1983) 'the stigma attached to women alcoholics' (Beckman, 1978) 'the female junkie' (Perry, 1979); and even 'women's abuse of food as a social disease' (Orbach, 1978). From these notions women are seen as users and abusers of a whole series of substances and they are portrayed as either out of control or in need of control, or both. These women researchers speculate that, unless these powerful images are confronted and indeed challenged, there is a danger that those responding to women in need of help (that is, the treaters) could perpetuate unknowingly myths and stereotypes harmful to the healing process.

From the previous chapter we already know that traditional discussions within the addiction field have focused primarily on substances which are 'mind-altering'. Reflecting on the content of these traditional discussions, we have seen that the terms 'addiction' or 'drug use' do not mirror adequately women's somewhat problematic relationship to substances, regardless of whether or not they may be 'mind-altering'. Also we have seen that we need expansive concepts and flexible theories inclusive of women.

Within the feminist debate on women's use of food, Orbach (1986, p. 24) argues quite convincingly that, as key features of anorexia, 'the starvation amidst plenty, the denial set against desire, the striving for invisibility versus the wish to be seen, are a metaphor for our age'. Furthermore women's problematic relationship with food may be seen as an excruciating spectacle in which women actually 'transform their bodies' in an attempt to deal with the contradictory requirements of the contemporary female role.

Given the above discussion, it appears that substance use, as a gender-illuminating notion, provides the necessary conceptual foundation upon which a women-oriented perspective can be built. Within the addiction field this notion helps to clarify outdated theoretical boundaries, which should be expanded if a full understanding of women and substance use is to become a reality. The underlying assumption here is that we cannot comprehend adequately the problems that women dependent on substances such as alcohol, prescribed drugs, illicit drugs, cigarettes and foods have without knowledge 'grounded in practical lived experience' (Stanley and Wise, 1983a). Therefore, within this vast area of social life, a feminist perspective as well as a clear, women-oriented response rooted in the identity and consciousness of women substance users are essential. This is a major strand of thinking highlighted throughout this chapter and indeed this text.

Let us now take a closer look at the way, for women, the notion of substance use, which implies varying levels of dependency on a variety of substances, can be linked with a general, feminist issue: dependency.

The 'unacceptable' and 'acceptable' faces of dependency

A very basic fibre of feminist thought is the idea that women, more than men, are socialised into dependency. As Graham (1983) suggests, the nature of dependency cannot be understood in isolation from either the sex–gender system or the process of capitalist expansion. In related contexts (Ettorre, 1989a, 1989b), the author has detailed the tandem definitions of 'dependency' and discussed, with special reference to the addiction field, the subtle implications of these dual meanings for women as a social group. To facilitate an understanding of these subtleties, we will develop below the initial ideas presented in those prior, related contexts.

Briefly, in its etymological roots, dependency stems from the Latin words 'de' and 'pendere', meaning to hang down from. However there are two meanings for dependence in common parlance, the word refering to either 'addiction' or 'a subordinate thing'. For women as a social group the former meaning is most definitely what I would call the unacceptable face of dependency, while the latter meaning is not only the acceptable face of dependency but also the prescribed norm for women. For example, dependency (of the 'addiction' kind) is socially 'unacceptable' when it interferes with a woman's social role as housewife, mother, dutiful daughter or female worker, while dependency (of the 'subordinate thing' kind) is seen to be good, highly valued or socially 'acceptable' when it involves being dependent on a husband, men, male protection or male superiors. With regard to its acceptable face, dependency is not only viewed as a fundamental part of any woman's life but it is the central operating principle in her life, her *raison d'être*. Gloria Steinem (1979, p. 66) has gone so far as to suggest that all women are 'male junkies'; that is, 'people who need regular shots of male-approval and presence both professionally and personally'.

While women who use substances, become depressed or 'go mad' can be seen as the casualties of a system which encourages dependence, their personal and social 'conditions' tend to make them even more dependent upon the patriarchal health care system. Two authors (Johnson and Auerbach, 1984), considering the direct effects of this health care system on women substance users, suggest that women's relationship to 'the three Ds' (doctors, dealers and darlings) create the greatest risks of addiction. In other words, 'the three Ds' are 'the persons, primarily men, who often lead them into addiction'.

In this specific context, Spender (1985) notes that, although women are used as they go through the 'caring' psychiatric system, they also use this system and in many instances become reliant upon it. Referring to the work of Phyllis Chesler, Spender says: 'The whole model of psychiatric help is "in character" for women . . . for while women are conditioned to find solutions in dependency then even greater dependence and self-abnegation can appear to be a plausible solution' (Spender, 1985, p. 145). For these women their 'dependent' status encourages further subservience.

On a more general level, this sensitive issue of dependency becomes more complex when we consider, as others have shown (Graham, 1983; Finch and Groves, 1982), that women's dependent status is contingent upon their being at the same time depended upon by others. For the majority of women, deeply involved in the social organisation of caring, giving care and helping others is a fundamental part of being a dependant. It is interesting to note here that, with special reference to the informal control of drinking in Finnish families, Holmila, Mustonen and Rannik (1990) suggest that the family's labour in preventing alcohol problems can be conceptualised as caring work. This illustrates quite clearly how complex the issue of dependency is within the private sphere.

Perhaps, in this light, we can see that in relation to women substance users the word 'dependency' has various shades of meanings on both a public/social and a private/individual level. This tells us that for a thorough enquiry into the women and substance use issue, key individual and social factors need to be highlighted. In other words we need to offer a full account of the day-to-day experiences of these women. My contention is that a vibrant analysis of the issue of women and substance use necessitates both a structural (social) and a processual (individual) explanation.

On the one hand, a processual approach which tends to focus primarily on the individual problems with 'dependence' (either of the 'subordinate thing' or 'addiction' kind) and/or on help seekers is quite limited. (See for example, Thom, 1984, 1986, 1987; Allan, 1987). Although this sort of approach helps us to get at subtle and often hidden, subjective meanings, this perspective remains uncritical and ahistorical. More specifically it is unable to explain fully the structural roots of power and for women, the issue of power (whether social, political or economic) is most important.

On the other hand, if a feminist approach is to develop in this area, clear links between the issue of women and substance use and the overall structural dynamics of power and dependency must be established. I use the term 'feminist approach' here because there is a world of difference between offering an analysis based on an uncritical acceptance of women's role, the gender arrangements, patriarchal power and so on and proposing explanations set in a women-oriented framework. It would be unwise for us to assume that any work on women and substance use is necessarily feminist simply because it focuses on women. If the central tenet upholds the image of women substance users as helpless 'victims', if we are unable to appreciate fully women's presence in this work or if the topic is introduced in distorted (that is, sexist) ways, the subordination of women remains unchallenged. Furthermore the gender order, with its established social division of patriarchy, is denied and perhaps, more significantly, the feminist notion that the private/female sphere is dependent on the public/male sphere (Garmarnikow *et al.*, 1983) is totally disregarded.

We need more work in this area 'by women and for women'. Links with this discussion will be made when we examine the notion of pleasure in the concluding section of this chapter. For our immediate purposes it is best to move on to look at ways in which a women-oriented methodology can be developed as a useful strategy in the production of feminist knowledge on substance use.

The development of a women-oriented methodology

The following discussion will focus on some of the advantages associated with viewing women and substance use as a feminist issue and, it is hoped, establish some pointers for future work in the area. If feminism is 'an attempt to insist upon the experience and very existence of women' (Roberts, 1981, p. 15) and if feminist is 'assuming a perspective in which women's experiences, ideas, and needs are valid in their own right' (Duelli-Klein, 1983), we need to be clear on the strategies we use to carry out research on women. Perhaps we could say that this demand for clarity arose in a more general context (social anthropology) when Ardener (1975) referred to both the complex 'technical' and 'analytical' issues, revolving around the category of 'women' in ethnographic work. However, regardless of our particular academic discipline, there are common practices which we share as we produce feminist knowledge. With reference to women and substance use, five interrelated problems need to be highlighted before we even begin to produce an environment open to this type of endeavour: the production of feminist knowledge.

First, traditional accounts tend to view women substance users as an 'homogeneous' social group without reference to key social factors such as age, ethnic origins, able-bodiedness, social class and sexual orientation. To challenge these accounts we need to expand both within and beyond established treatment settings, traditional research environments, 'taken for granted' social group-ings, particular academic disciplines and specific cultures. In other words, given that we live in societies more often than not characterised by inequalities in the gender order, we may want to assess how these inequalities affect our research and/or clinical practice. If we want to expand our work by focusing on specific groups of women, such as working-class women, black women/ women of colour, lesbian women or single women, we should examine social attitudes and practices furthering inequalities in the class system, institutionalised racism, heterosexism or social arrangements detrimental to single parents. While much social research has been done on the family, related research which emphasises the effects of women's substance use on the interplay between the public, primary sphere of social relations and the private, secondary female sphere of social relations would be fitting.

Within 'treatment' settings we may need to ask more questions than have been asked previously on how and why different sub-groups of women ask for help from already established networks of health care more often than other sub-groups of women. For example, in our health care system, is differential access to treatment for substance-abusing women in any way affected by social attitudes to class, race, age, ableness, sexual preference as well as to gender? How do different sub-groups of women such as elderly women, working-class women, black women, less able women, lesbian women, mothers and so on ask for help, and with what results? What about women who do not seek help? This leads us on to the second problem.

Traditional research in this area tends to focus on women already being processed in the treatment system or those seeking help (Annis and Liban, 1980). I would argue that this focus has distorted the image of women substance users. In other words the vertical relationships between the usual 'male treater' and the 'female treated' as well as between the researcher and the researched are emphasised to the obstruction of what Meis (1983) would term the 'view from below'. In this context I would share with Meis the conviction that this type of hierarchical research situation generates an acute distrust in the population of the 'researched'. It is only when our work is both actively captivated and captured by women's awarenesses, struggles and movements towards liberation that a view from below is possible. If we attempt to capture the 'researched''s needs and interests as an objective research desire, we create distortions as well as imposing a view from above.

Along with these strategies, we should become aware that any work in this area should be attempting to move away from looking at individual women who use substances. We need to uncover the collective experiences shared by women dependent on substances. If we continue to focus on solitary women, whether or not they are processed through the treatment system, we continue to perpetuate an individualist framework which does not allow us to understand why women pursue life styles that damage their health (Graham, 1990). This type of framework also removes the possibility of placing the issue of women and substance use within a political context.

Thirdly, as with those offering treatment to women problem drinkers in the United States (National Institute on Alcohol Abuse and Alcoholism, 1983), we need to offer a holistic approach, offering an insider's sensitivity to women's problems. With special reference to the overall provision for drug services, work in this area (MacGregor and Ettorre, 1987) has outlined the basic elements needed for a comparable approach, termed 'a pragmatic approach'. Reflecting strategies similar to the holistic approach, the pragmatic approach would begin to reform existing services to make them more flexible in response to special need groups (women, members of the black community and so on) as well as maintaining and developing forms of provision designed expressly and exclusively for specific groups such as women-only services.

Along with offering a holistic approach, we need to consider the benefits of self-help/mutual help groups as a forceful means of support for women. Seeing these groups as 'powerful resources for women in emotional distress and in the midst of oppressive life conditions', Belle (1984, p. 148) argues that within these groups women experience the awareness that they are not alone and, more importantly, that 'systemic rather than individual factors are responsible for many of their difficulties'. Perhaps, sharing Belle's sentiments, we are able to see this process as generating a powerful antidote to guilt and depression. This type of 'cure' is most certainly lacking in the field of substance use.

Fourthly, as conscientious scholars we need to consider ways of extending our analyses beyond traditional research settings and into wider social arenas. For example, Graham's (1987) study on women's smoking demonstrates quite effectively how the issue of women and substance use can be linked with wider health and welfare concerns such as poverty, single parenthood, family health and leisure. Additionally within the field of substance use the generation of a feminist perspective on women and dependency as well as a specific interest in the establishment of a framework sensitive to all types of women substance users, regardless of age, ethnic origins, preferred drug, sexual preference or social class, is beginning to be documented (Wolfson and Murray, 1987).

In this setting we may sense that doing feminist research, as Stanley and Wise (1983b) suggest, is really the 'doing of feminism' in a specific context. If one is a feminist, the doing of feminism is a matter of exposing the inherently political nature of every woman's life and this is a continuous process for all women. To generate this type of awareness and indeed practice in the field of addiction is difficult but possible and represents a major strategy in enlarging the limited scope of work carried out within this field. The fact that links between women's social position and women's use of substances are very rarely made in this area of research and clinical practice indicates the potential threat that 'doing feminism' currently poses.

Lastly, we need to challenge what can be referred to as the 'peopling of women'. This may be recognised as a familiar tactic, used in the addiction field as in others, resistant to a feminist analysis. For example, we often hear the phrase, 'women are people'. Sometimes this phrase is useful and other times it is not. It is useful for feminists when they need to demonstrate 'sameness' between men and women such as in the area of racial inequality or social disability. However one could argue that more often than not 'peopling women' is damaging for women. When one hears the term 'women are people too', one should be attentive. This may be a clever ploy, used by seemingly 'sympathetic' individuals. They may be disguising the fact that they are erasing women altogether from their analyses. For them, women are 'people' because they sense that a perspective on women would be too challenging or difficult to incorporate within their work. 'Peopling women' is a matter of wiping out women from analyses or subverting an understanding of women's position and, more importantly, paying lip service to the 'sameness' between men and women, while obscuring the crucial historical, political, economic and social differences which divide the sexes. The 'peopling of women' inevitably ends up with a general myopic vision in which women are totally out of focus.

The definition of people ignores all forms of social hierarchy, and male treaters and male theorists who refer to women as 'people' find their interests jeopardised by this type of exposé. If feminists are engaged in this 'dangerous' sort of 'doing', they may hear, uttered from the mouth of those in power, 'OK, talk about women and their problems but just remember they are people most of all.' My response is, 'It would be very useful if you stopped colonising the definition of people which obviously refers to white, middle-class men.' The field of substance use needs less 'peopling' of women and more 'doing' of feminism.

We have looked at the various problems which exist in the area of women and substance use as well as five strategies which are needed for the development of a women-oriented methodology. While serving as pointers for the future, these strategies suggest that our traditional research framework is capable of expansion and transformation through the adoption of a feminist perspective. In our concluding discussion, let us introduce the concept of pleasure into this arena and let us explore whether or not the introduction of this concept has any relevance for women as a social group.

Substance use and 'pleasure': is this relevant for women?

When the problems of women substance users are taken out of the private domain, society's experts more often than not fail to see the variety of reasons why women use drugs *differently* from men. Women's substance use and abuse may be seen as more of a social problem than men's because it implies 'destability' in the family. Specifically images of alcoholic women have been seen historically as a real threat to the clear lines between the gender roles of men and women (Appel, 1990). Furthermore there are few public settings, contexts or mechanisms whereby women can address their experiences in terms of the choices they make or the benefits they receive from their consumption of addictive substances. Underlying their substance use is the type of voluntary, active and creative use of drugs which one woman (Harpwood, 1982) describes and illustrates so well.

In the discussion of the concept of pleasure, readers must be very clear that the author is not advocating substance misuse. Rather it is suggested that we need to look perhaps more closely at the pleasurable effects of substances. In particular we need to ask ourselves why and how women experience their substance use as pleasurable and whether or not the use of substances can contribute to a woman's sense of well-being. A possible starting-point is the question: 'what pleases women?' Obviously to find an answer we need to preserve, as we saw from an earlier discussion in this chapter, a view from below.

We already know that the concept of pleasure for both men and women tends to be linked with sexual performance and pursuits and that, in this sexual arena, male sexual dominance is assumed to be natural (Holland, Ramazanoglu and Scott, 1990). However, as Griffin (1978) aptly states, 'It is said that women, exist for pleasure . . . Women are the weaker sex, it is said, and therefore, those women have survived who best succeeded in pleasing men.'

On the other hand, pleasure has other meanings that extend beyond the realm of the sexual. As Raymond (1986) suggests, pleasure for women includes the notion of empowerment. Similarly, Vance (1984) shows how pleasure and empowerment are linked particulary for those in a subordinate, social position: women. I would also suggest that women's investigation of pleasure is intrinsically related to, if not determined by, their specific material circumstances and life style choices (age, social class, sexual orientation, marital status, ethnic origins, psychological health, physical well-being, accommodation, number of dependents, paid employment and so on).

Given the above, pleasure for most women appears as a subverted or hidden reality. Visibility will be possible only if society changes to recognise women's needs, their integrity and their full human potential. As long as oppressive structures, related to the public expectation of dependency and the private sphere of domesticity, remain invisible, real pleasure will be denied for women. To break from these structures women need to become grounded in the positive dimensions of what Raymond (1986) calls 'their otherness'. That some women, as inhabitants of our stress-filled and drug-using society, turn to substances for pleasurable experiences could be an indication of this grounding process. For example, it has been suggested that, for women, 'taking drugs can be an attempt to meet our own needs' (DAWN, 1986). Do women turn to substances as a movement towards 'taking something for themselves' rather than giving and receiving pleasure as is the usual case? Here pleasure implies a certain amount of autonomy and assertiveness.

In the context of feminist theory, one author (Daly, 1984) contends that many women, because of their fragmented and isolated lives, accept the belief that happiness is attainable only after death. In an attempt to challenge this belief, Daly urges women to recognise that their quest for pleasure (what she terms 'lust for happiness') is, in the Aristotelian sense, a quest for a life of activity. In the highest sense this life of activity is contemplation or an activity of the mind. It should be noted that Daly is not proposing that all women should leave secular society and enter the reflective world of the cloister. Rather she is suggesting that 'women's whole, intellectual/passionate/sentient selves need to unfold' (Daly, 1984, p. 347) as women live and experience their daily lives in whatever situations they find themselves.

This distinctly feminist process demands that women become deeply aware of their creative powers, recognise their integrity as women and, most importantly, transcend 'patriarchal' patterns of thinking, speaking and acting. Through this process women begin to learn that real pleasure is linked with creativity and empowerment.

In the light of the discussions in this chapter, let us ask ourselves one question: what is on offer which allows the majority of women to focus energy on themselves, to be really autonomous or to actively create pleasure? In asking this question, we should be aware that women need more public and private space to explore what pleases them and to empower themselves as women. Specifically women substance users need to explore the many, often contradictory reasons why they turn towards and indeed use substances. They need to challenge stereotypical images which characterise them as diseased, neurotic, pathological, decadent or polluted. (For a detailed discussion of the notion of pollution *vis-à-vis* women's substance use, see Ettorre, 1989a.)

Perhaps, more importantly, women substance users need to search for alternative ways of preserving their integrity, exercising their autonomy and expressing their rage. As Connors (quoted in Daly, 1984, p. 358) demonstrates, women's sickness can be viewed as a way of directing women's potential 'deviance' (that is, defiance against patriarchy) away from a collective, public, structurally damaging path towards a somewhat private, professionally managed or individually manageable, self-destructive route. For example, experts view women alcoholics or problem drinkers as a diseased, sick or neurotic group who evidence what they refer to as the alcohol dependence syndrome. In reality these women may be evidencing a type of 'patriarchal defiance syndrome' as they keep their problem hidden in an environment of guilt and shame (Blume, 1990b).

In an illuminating critique on psychiatry, Rubin (1975, p. 146) suggests that for women the symptoms of neurotic behaviour (of which substance abuse is one) are symbolic expressions of the contradictions patriarchal society has imposed on them. Therefore these symptoms 'must be viewed with the utmost respect for their valid protest against the tyranny of women's condition'. The implication here is that what women say about themselves is not treated as consequential when it is treated as a symptom. In other words, if a woman is diagnosed as sick, whatever she says to her treater has little if any effect on removing this diagnosis. Furthermore the fact that 'women have protested with their lives . . . because they could not do otherwise' (Smith, 1975, p. 13) often remains invisible. For those women death was their ultimate act of defiance against a stigmatising society.

In a related context, Showalter (1985) exposed the fact that, during the latter part of the nineteenth century, the feminisation of insanity and the domestication of the lunatic asylums created a whole flock of specialists in 'female illnesses', such as hysteria and neurasthenia. Showalter also noted that the majority of asylums were overcrowded and most patients were women. Do we blink an eye when, from this feminist exposé, we discover that the disciplinary regime required within the asylums meant that the misuse of opiates and the practice of self-starvation (the precursors to modern-day addiction and anorexia) appeared to have been actively encouraged by the predominantly male 'experts'?

Today the asylums are gone, but women heroin addicts and anorexics remain. Notably there is a proliferation of more male specialists in 'female specialities', a growth which, in specific areas like reproductive technology and genetic engineering, exposes a patriarchal practice to 'undermine women's integrity and the struggle for women's liberation' (Spallone and Steinberg, 1987, p. 13). Nevertheless women have an autonomous way of making themselves, their collective pain and their struggles known throughout history. The fact that women heroin addicts and anorexics remain is a reflection, albeit faint, of this liberatory urge and pilgrimage of survival.

In conclusion, a basic contention of the discussion in this chapter has been that there is a need for a feminist perspective on women and substance use which moves beyond the established masculinist ways of thinking. We have also looked at substance use, dependency and pleasure as gender-illuminating notions in our attempt to map out a women-oriented perspective. If the issue of women and substance use is to be framed with this type of perspective, women substance users, 'expert' treaters and research scholars alike need to strive together to challenge images and practices which distort women's lives. We need to develop an acute, collective awareness that an ocean of energy, women's pleasure, should flow freely, neither hindered by outdated categories of thought and oppressive social practices nor inhibited by the debilitating effects of 'comforting' substances.

Perhaps, in this context, we could usefully ponder the words of Nor Hall (1980), as she reflects on the archetypal feminine. She says:

> Assembling and disassembling, remembering and dismembering, tearing apart and putting back together again the body of knowing: the moon, like the poppy flower, requires that your imagination enter into it in order to avoid the harm of possession . . . If you give a part of yourself to lunacy, she will permit you to pass to and from the realm of the moon's dark phase. Otherwise she will detain you. Stupor and blackness will possess you. (p. 65).

We all need symbols of conversion, yet there are no guidelines for rebirth, only meaningful transformations and the rhythm of becoming. Within this particular intellectual discourse, the process of change develops as moves to bring together pieces of the truth are made. Let us hope that, as the field of substance use becomes more sensitive to women, these changes will provide inner strength for women dependent on addictive substances to take a critical look at their substance use.

2

Women and alcohol

If I this oath maintain,
may I drink this glorious wine.
But if I slip or falter,
let me drink water. (Aristophanes, *Lysistrata*)

Introduction

In recent years evidence gathered on the increased prevalence of alcohol problems amongst women (Shaw, 1980; Ferrence, 1980; Alcohol Concern, 1988); the growing numbers of women problem drinkers seeking help (Wilson, 1976; Kent, 1981; NIAAA, 1983); the atypicality and relatively small numbers of women treated in specialist settings, particularly in the UK (Thom, 1984; Ettorre, 1985c) and the implied links between women's heavy drinking and stress (for example, Breeze, 1985; Snell, Belk and Hawkins, 1987) suggests that problem drinking amongst women has achieved status as a social problem as well as greater visibility as a women's issue.

Ahlstrom (1983) suggests that the women and alcohol issue has become important for three reasons: (1) the strong growth of alcohol consumption in western industrialised societies; (2) women's special role as an instrument of reproduction and an agent of socialisation; and (3) the rise of feminist research. While this type of view represents a minority opinion in the alcohol field, it does help to establish valuable pointers for the development of a feminist perspective on women and alcohol.

One of the main aims of this chapter is to provide the reader with a sense of the problems, conflicts and difficulties one confronts in defining women's relationship to alcohol as a feminist issue.

Developing a feminist perspective inevitably exposes a series of related problem areas, which include: the tension between the social sciences and the natural sciences within addiction research; the prioritisation of epidemiological methods to the detriment of clear sociological analyses; positivism versus critical social research; and social psychiatry as a legitimated social science versus women's studies as an acceptable, academic discipline. Perhaps most importantly the quest for a feminist perspective in this area reveals the existence of a sexist ideology, defining how women problem drinkers seeking help should feel and, in turn, be treated. This ideology tends to conceal the real needs and difficulties women with alcohol problems experience. This chapter seeks to illustrate how within a general view on women and substance use, a specific theory on women and alcohol can be developed.

In her discussion of the importance of feminist theory, Spender (1983, p. 1) suggests that, while both men and women have been involved traditionally in theory building, men are seen as *the* theorists. Men's theories as opposed to women's theories have been accepted as *legitimate*. In other words, 'only one sex owns the realm of theory'.

In the light of these comments, the reader should be aware that theory building in the alcohol field is fundamentally a male preserve. Traditionally male researchers and clinicians have had the power not only to define the women and alcohol issue but also to claim ownership of the problem over and above their female colleagues. Words like 'family', 'gender' and 'sex roles' tend to be used in an uncritical way, as taken-for-granted concepts. There is little if any effort made to link these concepts with important theoretical notions such as the sex–gender system, sexual discrimination, women's subordination and the social inequalities of sex, race and class. The following discussions begin to make these links and to take a first step in theory building for women in the alcohol field.

An appropriate starting-point for these discussions is to outline the key areas of concern covered in this chapter. In this way one begins to describe, understand and name women's experience with alcohol from a women-oriented point of view. The key areas of concern will focus on the resistance one encounters in viewing the woman and alcohol issue as a political issue; the double standard and the images of women problem drinkers; the effects of the definitions of alcoholism on alcohol-dependent women; discrimination in treatment and a women sensitive response to the foetal alcohol syndrome.

Viewing women and alcohol as a political issue

In a scholarly article entitled 'Historical and Political Perspective: Women and Drug Use', Edith Lisansky Gomberg (1982) asserts that the drug and alcohol issue for women is a 'political issue linked to gender roles, power, ambivalence and hidden angers and fears' in society. In making this assertion, Lisansky Gomberg moves towards an analysis that can be seen as women-oriented. She also contends that alcohol is 'the social drug' most widely used in contemporary society. Not surprisingly, most clinicians and researchers in the alcohol field would agree with her latter assertion, while taking issue with her former one. There are reasons for this type of conceptual discrimination. On the one hand, recognising the widespread use of alcohol is a basic operating principle in the alcohol field. On the other, providing grounds upon which the women and alcohol issue might be judged as political is seen as contentious. It is viewed as threatening to the *status quo*: the idea that a 'real alcoholic' is a man.

Theoretical resistance to establishing the women and alcohol issue as a feminist one is a very subtle, intellectual exercise. This theoretical resistance is supported by the general tendency to ignore overall social and political concerns, necessary for a full understanding of alcohol and its use in society. As a result, theories in the alcohol field tend to be apolitical and to legitimate inequalities based on sex, race and class.

Given that it is fairly uncommon to find discussions on the ideological and political significance of alcohol, there is a need to uncover significant 'structural' concerns if links are to be made between the women and alcohol issue and the politics of alcohol. For example, in the UK, consumers' expenditure on alcoholic drink was nearly £11 434 million in 1984 and this represented 7.5 per cent of all consumer expenditure (Royal College of General Practitioners, 1986). Work in the mid-1980s (Saunders, 1985) pointed out that as a nation Britain spends approximately £33 million on alcohol each day. The state makes approximately £5000 million a year from taxes on alcohol (Action on Alcohol Abuse, 1985).

The Central Policy Review Staff report (1979) which was not allowed to be published in this country and was eventually published in Sweden (Bruun, 1982) noted 16 government departments with direct interests in the alcohol trade. As Maynard (1985, p. 238) aptly states, 'no one in the Whitehall village has the designated role . . . to mobilise and implement an effective alcohol policy'. Besides the involvement of these government departments, a number of politicians, including such notables as Norman Fowler and Geoffrey Finsberg, have either direct or indirect interests in the alcohol industry (McConville, 1983). Regardless of politicians' varying interests in the alcohol industry, there are nine bars available for them on Whitehall's premises suggesting heavy drinking habits.

As far as the alcohol industry itself is concerned, it employs 3.4 per cent of all people employed in the UK and brewers and distillers as a group form more than 5 per cent of the Stock Exchange's total equity market (Thurman, 1983). The alcohol drinks trade reports that 10 per cent of expenditure on advertising has some effect on demand, while they cannot identify which 10 per cent (Maynard, 1985). Significantly there is a glaring imbalance between the expenditure on alcohol advertising and sponsorship (estimated at £150 million a year) and the alcohol budget of the Health Education Council – now the Health Education Authority (approximately £200 000 a year) (Royal College of General Practitioners, 1986).

There is a $170 billion a year global alcohol market, dominated by 27 major multinational corporations, each of which have annual sales exceeding $1 billion and with branches in eight major industrialised nations (Cavanagh and Clairmonte, 1985). During the economic recession of the late 1970s, British multinationals were forced to expand and create new markets both at home and abroad. Markets were sought in the third world, while domestic market growth was generated through the development of alcohol sales in multiple retail chain stores such as Marks and Spencer, Sainsburys, Tesco, Safeways and International Stores, a subsidiary of British American Tobacco. Alcohol became available at lower retail prices and by 1977 approximately half of Britain's supermarkets had licences to sell alcohol (Otto, 1981).

In recent years, Sainsburys and Marks & Spencers have been included among the eight powerful companies which control 40 per cent of the UK's wine distribution (Maynard, 1985). One major consequence of this development has been that women consumers are increasingly the target of producers and retailers.

While profit from alcohol consumption appears to take priority over public health, anyone suffering from individual problems related to alcohol consumption is labelled a 'misuser'. In particular women are affected, not only by being prime targets for 'new-style' alcohol marketing strategies but also by being seen as out of control, a social threat, sexually permissive, destructive and endangering their family's stability and well-being if they develop an alcohol problem. Perhaps, more significantly, if drink helps to release a woman's anger or bitterness for whatever reason, she is seen as dangerous or aggressive (O'Donohue and Richardson, 1984). Regardless of these condemnations, women are less likely to receive treatment if seeking comfort in a bottle gets a little out of hand (White, 1984).

Alcohol Concern (1988) reports that, with the whole nation drinking more, women, in common with men, are experiencing more drink-related problems. While it is estimated that 2 per cent of the female adult population has a drinking problem, the majority of female heavy drinkers are unmarried and under 25 or married but without children at home. While women tend to drink less than men, their drinking is increasing with greater spending power. The result is higher levels of harm (Alcohol Concern, 1987).

Between 1979 and 1984, female deaths from chronic liver disease and cirrhosis rose 9 per cent . Female admissions to mental hospitals for alcohol misuse rose 60 per cent between 1977 and 1986 (Alcohol Concern, 1988). In the United States the overall mortality rate from alcoholism is greater for women than it is for men. Furthermore the death rate for female alcoholics is estimated at 2.7 to seven times that of non-alcoholic women (Cyr and Moulton, 1990).

What must be remembered here is that the problems women experience with alcohol tend to be mediated through their intimate partnerships with men. Women are more likely than their male counterparts to become heavy drinkers in response to psychological stress (Allan and Cooke, 1986) and female stress is most likely linked with relationships. As Morgan (1987, p. 129) suggests, 'the effects and characteristics associated with alcoholic beverages have been used symbolically and instrumentally to promote systems of subordination and domination' linked with race, class and sex. She contends further that women have experienced 'systematically pervasive, symbolic and substantive domination in relation to alcohol'. In a real sense, as one author contends (Room, 1983, p. 263), alcohol is so pervasive and is applicable to so many public and private issues that 'it is a wonderful tool for outlining and illuminating the structure of our societies'.

The double standard and the images of women problem drinkers

Women's experience of personal stress and social subordination are not the only factors which can be seen to highlight the women and alcohol issue. Racism, classism, ageism, heterosexism and every other system of inequality that erodes women's power, their courage, their integrity and their self esteem 'serve to contribute to their drinking problems, perpetuate them and intensify their painful effects' (Sandmair, 1980, p. 242). For women, problem drinking is highly disgraceful and, perhaps not surprisingly, it has been described as 'deviant deviance' (Allan and Cooke, 1986).

There is no doubt that women problem drinkers present a direct challenge to social stereotypes and culturally defined expectations of 'normal' acceptable women (Fillmore, 1984a, 1984b). They face a whole variety of problems rooted in their position as women in society, particularly if they seek help for their drinking problem (Beckman and Amaro, 1984; Beckman, 1984). Furthermore, while drinking, especially problem drinking, is seen to contradict social ideals of feminine behaviour (Rosett and Weiner, 1984), it has been suggested that alcoholic women go so far as to violate all cherished ideals of contemporary feminism (Crisp, 1984). In effect women problem drinkers experience a variety of problems of living or what Murphy and Rosenbaum (1987) refer to as 'polyproblems'. These 'polyproblems' do not allow women problem drinkers to fit comfortably within society or the alcohol treatment system.

Regardless of whether or not women drink, all women share the same cultural commandment to be the guardians of moral and social values (Youcha, 1978). While this commandment has been preserved over the ages by men, women's role has been equated with the stabilising function of wife and mother. Women with drinking problems present a special threat to this traditional female role and are considered to have deserted respectability in every area of their lives. Since there is a greater chance that moral judgements will be made about women who drink excessively than about men who are heavy drinkers (Litman, 1978), a double standard is operating. Clearly, in relation to men, women alcoholics tend to experience a stigma that is more distressing and more destructive than that suffered by men.

A powerful medium that has helped to shape this distorted representation of women alcoholics in contemporary society has been film. In this context the stigma associated with alcoholism in women is very clear and alcoholic women are portrayed as lonely, unhappy, lacking self-confidence, destructive and dependent (Harwin and Otto, 1979).

Along with the stigma attached to women alcoholics is the notion that a woman who drinks is sexually promiscuous. In fact drunkenness in women 'is not simply associated but equated with rampant sexuality' (Sandmair, 1980, p. 14). Sometimes links are made between women's alcoholism and prostitution. As one author (Lisansky Gomberg, 1982) points out, prostitution for these women is a 'source of income' rather than evidence of unbridled sexuality. Others (Silbert, Pines and Lynch, 1982) link prostitution and substance use (including alcohol) as the 'behavioural translation' of these women's 'endless cycles of victimization' as well as expressions of their self-destructiveness.

On the one hand, a woman with a drinking problem does not need to be a prostitute to have a promiscuous image. She is promiscuous by the very fact that she is a drinker. On the other, a prostitute who drinks is perhaps pitied more than her 'non-prostituting' sister. As an alcoholic, the prostitute is seen as doubly promiscuous: because of her drink and because of her type of sex/work.

In certain societies or in specific social situations, drunkenness defines a 'real man'. For women this is not true. Society expects that women be in control of themselves on most, if not all, occassions and, in some well-defined social contents, in control of their husband's drinking as well as their own (Holmila, 1985). Social expectations are clear: women should not get drunk in public or, indeed, display any type of drunken behaviour. There is a real social stigma attached to a woman who drinks too much. A woman alcoholic is seen to be in private a bad mother, uncaring for her children, or an irresponsible wife, not considering the needs of her husband. In public she is viewed as unforgivably out of control of her domestic and/or work situation or as an evil or loose woman who cannot be trusted.

One author (Cohen, 1981) contends that established stereotypes such as the suburban housewife who is bored and frustrated, and the menopausal woman, living in an empty nest, are based on valid observations. While adding the liberated young college girl and the harassed woman executive to the list of stereotypes, this author suggests further that women are adapting a masculine type of drinking behaviour. A similar way of thinking is put forward by Robertson and Heather (1986) who propose not only that women have much greater freedom, including the freedom to drink, but also that the stigma attached to women's drinking has largely disappeared.

The major effect of these arguments is to devalue, whether consciously or not the women and alcohol issue as a feminist concern. It appears that to increase the stereotypes of the women alcoholic is to produce an image of the liberated drinking woman. This image reflects the *status quo* or a male view of the world. In effect this type of thinking conceals the reality of the lives of women drinkers. There is a need for less rather than more stereotypes of women with alcohol problems. An awareness of the women and alcohol issue which is women-centred as well as women-defined needs to be generated further. As Sandmair (1980, p. 242) aptly states, 'If female drinking problems are increasing, it is most likely not because women's liberation has arrived but because it has not.' While times have changed, social attitudes towards the woman alcoholic have remained the same. They have been consistently stigmatising and isolating. Characterised by polystereotypes, women alcoholics have been defined as having polyproblems.

The alcohol dependence syndrome and alcohol dependent women

Traditionally the alcohol field has been dominated theoretically by the medical profession, particularly psychiatrists. Although psychiatrists are intrinsically natural scientists, some 'alcohol psychiatrists', such as Edwards (1977, 1980, 1982), Glatt (1974, 1975), Madden (1979) and Vaillant (1983), do lend support to the social scientific point of view. However, given that psychiatrists are not generally known for incorporating feminist analyses into their work, the needs of women alcoholics have been consistently ignored in general formulations on alcoholism. Not surprisingly, as the basis for modern-day medical thinking on alcoholism, the 'disease concept of alcoholism', proposed by Jellinek (1952, 1960) focuses almost exclusively on the 'male alcoholic'.

In recent years the disease concept of alcoholism has been disguised and translated into the 'alcohol dependence syndrome' (Edwards and Gross, 1976). The alcohol dependence syndrome is viewed as a complex psycho-physiological disorder which, as Heather (1985) points out, is essentially a disease-oriented and medically based conception of problem drinking. It is interesting to note that the dependence used in the phrase 'alcohol dependence syndrome' refers to dependence of the addiction kind rather than dependence of the subordinate thing kind. No male or female theoretician in the alcohol field has ever talked about a male dependence syndrome. For example, that men, whether problem drinkers or not, are dependent in the private sphere on women carers for familial, social and sexual servicing is not a topic for discussion. To some this may be surprising, given that the medical profession's attraction to and use of syndrome categories to describe social problems is such that scientific considerations have sometimes been suspended (Chick, 1985). Suggesting male dependence on women in the ways mentioned above would perhaps be seen as offering a type of feminist analysis of this social problem. In the eyes of the medical profession, this might be viewed as suspending scientific discourse in the field.

The main problems which exist with current definitions of alcoholism and the alcohol dependence syndrome are that drinking problems tend to be viewed as individual, behavioural or physiological problems. The experts and research scientists are more concerned with 'causes' or etiological explanations and 'disease patterns' or epidemiological issues than with issues of social inequality. Generally these concerns serve the interests of the medical profession, keep them theoretically in power and allow traditional ideas to go unchallenged. Of course, if and when women are mentioned, they are usually seen as an appendage to men within the family structure where women are seen to belong (Orford and Edwards, 1977). On closer analysis, wives of alcoholics are seen as acting out masochistic behaviour, while alcoholic women are seen to have a greater destructiveness than male alcoholics (Glatt, 1974).

Explanations of alcoholism, whether in the form of the disease concept of alcoholism or the alcohol dependence syndrome, were created out of a need to deal with alcohol misuse primarily in clinical populations. These explanations have served to prioritise treatment and rehabilitation issues. As a result serious discussions around any social, economic and political issue related to problem drinking in *both* non-clinical and clinical populations have been absent in the field. Specifically, for women with alcohol problems, fundamental issues such as domestic stress, violence in the family, sex role conflict, recreational drug use, the heterogeneity of women as a social group, the need for a gender-sensitive perspective and a discussion of women's 'polyproblems' remain hidden if not ignored.

In another context the author has outlined the problems related to the alcohol field as being multidisciplinary and 'multisexist' (Ettorre, 1986a). The view was put forward that alcohol sociology as 'drunken sociology' exists because many alcohol sociologists have been either 'sex blind' (that is, they ignore women's experience of alcohol) or 'double blind' (that is, they ignore the complex interplay between sex, gender and social practice). As a result what emerges from social theories on alcohol proposed by male theorists, whether psychiatrists or sociologists, is the assumption that alcoholism is a 'man's disease' or a 'male problem'. This overriding assumption hinders the development of a perspective which offers 'a social structural framework for examining women's problematic behaviour in terms of traditional gender roles and relationships' (Valentich, 1982, p. 17).

Furthermore the subtle resistance to this type of gender-sensitive perspective will continue until misconceptions of problem drinking are challenged and replaced by notions reflective of real social and political processes. An analysis of women's unease with 'dependence of the subordinate thing kind' needs to be included in any theoretical formulation of women's addiction to alcohol, her 'dependence of the addiction kind'. For example, as Turner (1987, p. 2) contends, disease is viewed as a 'neutral and natural entity residing in nature' (the body of the patient). He suggests that this concept needs to be criticised by the use of a more holistic notion, social embodiment. This latter sociological notion allows us to see more closely how the split between the mind and body, upheld by the medical profession, conceals important political divisions in society. Furthermore this mind and body split tends to separate the individual from society. It has served not only to subordinate a satisfactory medical sociology but also to subvert the need for a feminist analysis.

Given the above, the alcohol field needs a sociology of the body in the same way that feminism needs a theory of pleasure (Vance, 1984). If the notion of social embodiment is taken seriously in the alcohol field, theoreticians will need to look more carefully than in the past at the way alcohol use and abuse affects the body politic. They will 'need to examine how alcohol as representing morality or immorality and power and weakness' (Morgan, 1987) interacts with our natural milieu, our bodies. These bodies are 'natural' sites which allow individuals in society to have both moral and social agency. Nevertheless theoreticians will need to be aware that, given the current inequalities in society, moral and social agency have different implications for men and women as social groups.

It is not appropriate in this context to discuss further the nature of social embodiment as it effects women and the reader is directed to debates on this issue within feminist theory (Butler, 1987; Harding and Hintikka, 1983; Chodorow, 1978). What is important in this discussion is to point out that within the disease concept of alcoholism as well as the updated disease conception, the alcohol dependence syndrome, alcoholic women fare worse than alcoholic men. To assume that women alcoholics are 'worse' or 'more deviant' than men alcoholics implies that the consciousness of theoreticians and treaters making these unsubstantiated assumptions needs to be raised before women alcoholics gain equal treatment, whether institutional or not in relation to men.

Seeking help and finding discrimination

As we have seen, within the alcohol field women's polyproblems, their situations and their needs have been largely unacknowledged within the research world. We already know from previous discussions in this book that research on women and substance misuse has been referred to as a 'non-field' (Kalant, 1980).

In the last 20 years there has been a spate of both individual and collective attempts, particularly by women (and sympathetic men) alcohol researchers and clinicians to alter misconceptions about women alcoholics and to include this group firmly within the alcohol field. (See, for example Lisansky, 1957; Wood and Duffy, 1966; Kinsey, 1966, 1968; Pemberton, 1967; Curlee, 1968, 1969, 1970; Schuckit *et al.* 1969; Sclare, 1970; Rathod and Thomson, 1971; Jones, 1971; Lindbeck, 1972; Parker, 1972; Gomberg, 1974, 1976; Beckman, 1975; Greenblatt and Schuckit, 1976; Morgan and Sherlock, 1977; Mulford, 1977; Burtle, 1979; Kalant, 1980; Camberwell Council on Alcoholism, 1980; Corrigan, 1980; National Institute on Alcohol Abuse and Alcoholism, 1980; Wilsnack and Beckman, 1984; *Journal of Psychoactive Drugs*, 1987; Cooke and Allan, 1984; Litman, 1986; Fillmore, 1987; Thom, 1987 and Harrison and Belille, 1987; Blume 1990a, 1990b; Kent, 1990.) Unfortunately much of the above-mentioned work has focused on clinical populations. 'Sex differences in treatment outcome' appear to be the key words in these types of presentations. Nevertheless this work has been important in establishing valuable pointers for those working in the field. Specifically work exposing the existence of male bias (Vanicelli and Nash, 1984) and the sexist assumption that women are no different from their male counterparts (Richmond, 1981) emerged from this tradition.

Other research in this treatment tradition suggested that alcoholic women suffer from lower self-esteem, more anxiety and a greater sense of powerlessness and inadequacy about their drinking behaviour than alcoholic men (Beckman, 1978, 1980). The problems of an alcoholic woman are often times compounded when she is judged by society's standards of what is an 'acceptable' women and meets with disapproval instead of compassion when she seeks help (Rosett and Weiner, 1984).

The literature on women and alcohol tends to suggest that women use alcohol as an avenue for relieving the stresses, discomforts and strains of daily life (Reed, 1985, 1987; Knupfer, 1982; Cuskey, Berger and Densen-Gerber, 1977; Snell, Belk and Hawkins, 1987). A study on Canadian women (Philo, Murdoch, Lapp and Mariner, 1986) reported that alcohol use in women is related to such reasons as 'relaxation', 'to forget' and 'to forget cares due to tension'. In all of these studies the problems of alcoholic women or women's use of alcohol are linked whether implicitly or explicitly to women's subordinate role in society. Lisansky Gomberg and Gomberg (1984, p. 250) have observed that two variables, depression and sex-role conflict, have been used as 'explanations of female alcoholism or at least primary antecedent events and they have dominated the literature on female alcoholism'. In turn these authors stress the need for those concerned about women alcoholics to look closely at other variables such as social isolation, anger, work role, marital role and parental role.

While problem drinking for women has been associated with family life (Estep, 1987) and marital problems (Lindbeck, 1972), other researchers (Hatsukami and Owen, 1982) found that performing multiple roles (wife, mother *and* worker) helped to serve as a protection against relapse for women alcoholics. Within the realm of treatment it has been suggested that both men and women with abundant interpersonal networks found these networks to be important resources during the rehabilitation process. Of course in this context we must be aware that men have more access to social networks beyond the domestic sphere and that women's networks tend to be named, defined and controlled by men (Raymond, 1986).

In the light of this discussion, one author Stephenson (1980, p. 12) contends that we must not be 'seduced' by theories which present only an 'individual and intrapsychic basis for problems'. On the contrary, this author contends that treaters need to help women alcoholics become aware that, as women belonging to a specific social group, their problems mirror the inequalities experienced by all women. For this particular group of women, their problems of living are 'not neurotic' and are often 'confused with psychiatric disorders'. Before treaters become aware of these issues, they need to recognise the special treatment needs of women (MacLennan, 1976) and 'develop services for an undercatered for and stigmatised group' (Waterson and Ettorre, 1989, p. 124).

While there are many problems that are evident within existing treatment systems, an extensive literature review on treatment effects for women problem drinkers outlines clearly the basic requirements needed to move forward (Duckert, 1984). That alcohol treatment and counselling services are often sexist (Murphy and Rosenbaum, 1987), orientated towards men (Reed, 1987; DAWN, 1985c) and insensitive to the needs of black women (Jenkins Gaines, 1976; Corrigan and Anderson, 1982; Nolan and

Day, 1988; Peckham Black Women's Group, 1985) as to well as lesbians (Hawkins, 1976) suggests that new components need to be included within existing services if they are to be sensitive to the needs of all different groups of women. To attract women to services demands that 'women-friendly' services be developed. In a study of recruitment to alcohol treatment, Duckert (1988) points out that women were reluctant about undergoing official treatment because of adverse consequences (that is, the stigma attached to being in treatment and losing their children). Developing 'women-friendly' services may imply the need to consider women only services.

An exploration of the need for women only services can be seen as important in moving towards the creation of services visibly sensitive to women (Jessup and Green, 1987). In arguing for a feminist psychotherapy for the treatment of women alcoholics, Connor and Babcock (1980) suggest that until sexism is recognised and worked through from all angles of these women's experiences (including treatment), sexism will continue to exist as a fuel for their 'pathology'.

Interestingly enough, in Britain the Royal College of Psychiatrists (1986, p. 160) devotes a paragraph of their report, *Alcohol: Our Favourite Drug*, to the need for treatment programmes to accommodate women's specific needs. Neighbourhood-based clinics and the provision for creches were viewed as important considerations for women. It has been some time since the production of this report and the needs of women with drink problems have still to be accommodated.

A women-sensitive approach to the foetal alcohol syndrome

In recent years there has been a growing concern about the effects of alcohol on the foetus and the term 'foetal alcohol syndrome' (FAS) was coined in a 1973 *Lancet* article entitled 'Recognition of the foetal alcohol syndrome in early infancy' by K. L. Jones and D. W. Smith (1973). Since that time there has been a growth of medical research in this area and one author (Rosett, 1980, p. 642) noted that 'clinical observations on over 245 cases of FAS have been reported from medical centres around the world'. It is generally the case that the most stigmatised female alcohol user is the pregnant woman (Jessup and Green, 1987), but there has been very little work in the alcohol field which examines the social implications of FAS or asks whether or not the emergence of this syndrome is a political issue as well as a distinct, medical syndrome. The clinical syndrome, 'nutmeg intoxication', has also been identified in pregnant women (Lauy, 1987) who experience an acute anticholinergic overstimulation. Perhaps analysing the reasons for the creation of these clinical syndromes is more of a feminist issue than meets the eye? For example, what substance will be next on the list of substances to be avoided by pregnant women? What substance will be used further to put women under surveillance and to stigmatise women substance users, particularly if they are pregnant?

In this context it is important to note that medical opinion on the use of alcohol by pregnant women is divided (Alcohol Concern, 1988) and research findings in this area remain inconclusive (Hingson, 1985). The primary research findings which suggest predictors of foetal harm are those studies related to smoking and pregnancy (Kline, Stein and Hutzler, 1982; Hingson, 1985). Plant's (1985) study on drinking during pregnancy found that moderate levels (less than 10 units of alcohol per week) did not result in foetal harm. Yet extreme caution was evidenced in Australia's 'Pregnant Pause' campaign directed at pregnant women, who were told to stop drinking (Healy, 1980).

Despite the lack of consensus in the field the following comments and observations tend to dominate discussions in this area:

> It's better to be safe than sorry . . . Women are best advised to cut out drinking completely even if they are just considering getting pregnant. (Robertson and Heather, 1986)

> The consensus is that responsible advice today must be that women should aim not to drink during pregnancies. (Griffith Edwards, quoted in CIBA Foundation, 1984)

> In the 1970's medics called fetal alcohol or maternal alcohol consumption the leading known cause of mental retardation in the Western world. (Hingson, 1985)

Prior to these comments, Gomberg writing within a feminist perspective (1979) had already noted that, whether or not women are at risk during pregnancy, they are stigmatised by the body of literature on the foetal alcohol syndrome. Generally all pregnant women substance users are under the 'tyranny of the foetus' (Pollitt, 1990) and increasingly monitored by medical authorities and in some instances the law (ISDD, 1990; Roberts, 1990; Fortney, 1990; Jopke, 1990). Priest (1990) suggests that, while not drinking is a pregnancy ritual of the late 1980s, abstinence from alcohol during this time has all the trappings of a taboo. This author asks whether the alcohol taboo keeps women from dangerous actions or creates the perception of danger where none exists. Simply, is the taboo about reality or control of women? The answer is that it is about both.

For example, few scientists in the field discuss the fact that testicle shrinkage (testicular atrophy) occurs amongst men who are heavy drinkers (Morgan and Pratt, 1982; Robertson and Heather, 1986). Men drinkers, as a social group, consume more alcohol and have heavier drinking levels than women. Thus far a body of literature advising male heavy drinkers to stop drinking altogether or to risk testicular atrophy is non-existent. Clearly, as has been suggested previously (Smart and Smart, 1978), women's sexuality is viewed as needing more control than men's. Moreover the message of the FAS literature is the need to control women's sexuality as well as the prevention of foetal harm.

When the FAS argument is used not only to stigmatise women drinkers more than they have been hither to but also to suggest that women are less responsible than men, a double standard can be seen to exist. The implication is that women's alcohol use is in need of more control and surveillance by the medical profession. Rosett and Weiner (1980, p. 148), focusing on the role of the medical profession say: 'The interest and concern of those to whom the pregnant woman has turned for health care are powerful forces for reducing her alcohol consumption and protecting her foetus.' Rosett (1980, p. 644) revised this statement: 'The knowledge, together with the interest and concern of those to whom the pregnant woman has turned for health care, is a powerful force for improving her health and that of her unborn child.' If interest, concern and knowledge are 'powerful forces', from where does the power come or, simply, who gives the power? Are women during pregnancy incapable of protecting their own bodies and foetuses or improving their own health? Is dependence on the holders of these powerful forces, presumably doctors, so complete that these women are unable to produce healthy children without doctors' interest, concern and knowledge? Perhaps, more significantly, how can a 'child' be 'unborn', as the above authors suggest?

If women were properly informed of the real risks of heavy drinking during pregnancy and if adequate resources were spent on providing accurate health promotion campaigns in the area of drinking and pregnancy, those uttering statements similar to the ones quoted above would attempt to offer to women more substance and less polemics.

There is no doubt that there is a link between heavy drinking and abnormal babies. Unlike other problems associated with substance abuse in pregnancy, FAS appears to be a clinically observable entity with specific characteristics for diagnosis (Smith and Smith, 1990). However, linked to the medical profession's concern and interest in the FAS, there is the distinct process by which pregnancy has become highly medicalised and increasingly 'pathologised'. This phenomenon can be set against the background of the general mobilisation of the medical profession around women's wombs which, as Oakley (1984) contends, have been 'captured'. One woman gynaecologist (Savage, 1986) has indicated that medical interventions during pregnancy have occurred without good scientific evidence that they are necessary and that pregnancy tends to be accepted more as an illness than a normal life event. In effect women's reproductive powers are taken away from them as they become increasingly dependent on symptoms, syndromes and diagnoses made by male doctors during the course of their pregnancies. This process mirrors developments in other areas of the medical profession where, under the guise of a benevolent concern, doctors and scientists continue to use reproductive technologies to appropriate women's reproductive power (Corea, 1985; Corea et al., 1985; Spallone and Steinberg, 1987; Spallone, 1989).

Nevertheless there is a notable absence of criticism about the FAS particularly by women researchers and clinicians in the alcohol field. It is generally accepted on face value. This is perhaps surprising given the elaborate debates developing around the new reproductive technologies and the issue of foetal rights (Gallager, 1987) within the area of women's studies. In this context a statement such as 'the pregnant drinker [referring to a woman] is actually two clients: the mother and the fetus' (Little and Ervin, 1984, p. 182) has profound ethical implications for women.

If we assume, as the above authors imply, that the foetus (as a client) has 'personhood', we will also have to assume that a women who harms this 'person' through drinking is grossly negligent. She is seen as guilty of a double abuse: to herself and to this child/person inside her. However it becomes clear that with the FAS argument, the foetus takes priority over the pregnant woman. Additionally, if the foetus dies because of a woman's heavy drinking, the potential charge of 'manslaughter' or 'second degree murder' may well be used. Of course there are legal and ethical considerations which would affect any judicial decision-making process. Here the key issue is that, if one argues for foetal rights rather than reproductive rights, one ignores the actual needs of pregnant women, regardless of whether or not they are drinking. There is a need to see clearly the links between the issues of foetal rights, the foetal alcohol syndrome and the vested interests of the medical profession in keeping pregnant women under increasing surveillance and control.

It should be noted that the above discussion is not meant to promote more than moderate drinking during pregnancy. In fact the general consensus is that pregnant women are able to safely consume one absolute ounce of alcohol a day. (This is the equivalent of four glasses of wine or two pints of beer.) Risks for pregnant women who drink heavily are involved, but these risks have been known to exist since the 1800s. It is only recently, within the past 20 years, that the medical profession has taken up this issue.

Nevertheless there is a need to expose some of the hidden, feminist issues which are involved in discussions of the foetal alcohol syndrome. Exposing these issues reveals that the women and alcohol issue has profound effects both on women's public and their private lives. The fact that the FAS issue has become more visable as a women's issue since the 1970s and that there is considerable media attention given to the FAS is worthy of concern and serious attention.

The mixture of the alcohol dependence syndrome, the foetal alcohol syndrome and women can be seen perhaps more as a poison than as a dangerous social cocktail. This poisonous mixture is ever so slowly destroying a pregnant woman's right to take responsibility for her own body and her own drinking practices.

Empowerment, the antidote, can only be effective if and when women sense that their well-being and that of their *future* children is in their own hands.

In this area it could be argued that women need more social agency rather than a greater imposition of moral agency by 'moral agents'. It was implied earlier in this chapter that resistance to a feminist perspective on alcohol will continue until the disease notion/alcohol dependence syndrome is challenged and replaced by theories sensitive to both women and men. To begin this process is to challenge some of the issues surrounding the foetal alcohol syndrome. If the FAS is being used against women, this needs to be exposed. Constructive ways forward are needed to educate women if they are being abused under the guise of the FAS.

In conclusion, the main aim of this chapter has been to look at some of the problems which arise when we look at the women and alcohol issue within a feminist context. We have seen that theoretical formulations offered in this field tend to be apolitical and individualistic. Within these formulations resistance to a women-sensitive perspective is evident.

The discussions in this chapter have emerged from a conscious attempt to understand and *to name* women's experience of alcohol from a feminist point of view. That 'polyproblems' and 'polystereotypes' exist more for women alcoholics than men alcoholics, that a double standard is perpetuated in the field; that the disease concept of alcoholism or the alcohol dependence syndrome further stigmatise women alcoholics, that women seeking help encounter discrimination and that the unquestioning acceptance of the foetal alcohol syndrome presents a direct threat to women's reproductive rights indicate an overwhelming need to expand the current debates about women which exist in the alcohol field.

Researchers need to look beyond clinical populations. Both clinicians and researchers need to educate themselves about the politics of alcohol *use and misuse* and the effects of these politics on women. Most importantly, the disgrace that is linked to women's misuse of alcohol needs to be challenged and powerful stigmas removed. In time, it is hoped, a perspective which offers an ample framework for examining the problems women experience in terms of traditional gender roles and relationships will be developed in the alcohol field. Finally women alcoholics of whatever age, sexual orientation, social class and race need to reclaim their lost power: to name their experiences from an awareness of what it means to be a woman in a society that brands them as outcasts.

3

Women and minor tranquillisers

He won't explain to you what's wrong
He'll give you a lecture ten minutes long
A case of hysterical fear
Is your problem my dear
Take these pills and come back in a year
What can you do surgery blues
Don't take such an interest
Doctor knows best . . .

('Surgery Blues' by the Stepney Sisters quoted on the cover of *Women's Health Handbook: A Self-Help Guide* compiled by Nancy MacKeith)

Introduction

Psychotropic drugs comprise one of the most commonly prescribed categories of drug in industrialised countries and over the years, the frequent usage of these drugs has become a matter of concern for research scientists in a variety of fields.

In assessing this issue on an international scale, medical experts (Idanpaan-Heikkila, Ghodse and Khan, 1987) have suggested that if psychotropic drug use is to be understood and indeed effective health and social policies be developed, it is essential that the abuse potential of these drugs, their liability to induce dependence and the possible social and public health consequences be thoroughly investigated.

In Britain specific attention over the past decade has tended to focus on the use of minor tranquillisers (benzodiazepines) with the established medical view that their use should be as a temporary measure of symptomatic relief (Committee on the Review of Medicines, 1980). New prescribing guidelines, issued by the

Committee on the Review of Medicines (1988) and supported by the Royal College of Psychiatrists (1988) recommended prescribing tranquillisers for a maximum of four weeks with the proviso that this be viewed only as a last measure of treatment.

A general consensus amongst those working in the field has been that basic data on the patterns and prevalence of psychotropic drugs illuminate psychotropics as 'social drugs', similar to alcohol (Cooperstock and Parnell, 1982) with important social, behavioural and public health implications. Given this broad conceptual framework, social scientists working in the field have had a valuable role to play in mapping out the social meanings of psychotropic drug use (Cooperstock and Lennard, 1986), investigating the consultation process in which prescriptions are given (Raynes, 1979, 1980) and specifically in providing information on the drug users, their health status and social characteristics (Riska and Klaukka, 1984).

This chapter will begin to develop a feminist analysis of the prescription of psychotropic drugs to women, specifically minor tranquillisers or benzodiazepines and we will focus on key social issues related to women's use and misuse of these psychotropic substances. While most 'addictive' substances tend to be self-administered, the issue of women's addiction to benzodiazepines is particularly interesting. These substances are most commonly mediated through a doctor who provides patients with their first prescription. If prescriptions are offered on a repeat basis, pharmacological addiction will inevitably follow.

It has been suggested that benzodiazepine-containing drugs have become the most controversial class of medicines used to treat mental disorders (DuPont, 1990). These drugs came on to the world 'legal' drugs market in the early 1960s and by the mid-1960s their usage had begun to increase rapidly. Brand-names of some of the more well known drugs include: Librium, Valium, Ativan, Mogadon, Serenid, Halcion, Frisium and Normison. As demand for minor tranquillisers increased and prescriptions continued to grow, benzodiazepines became a popular drug, used widely by many general practitioners.

In her book, *The Tranquilliser Trap and how to get out of it*, Joy Melville (1984, p. 7) argues that minor tranquillisers were the restorative – the nearest thing to bottled happiness you could get – and they were used to combat stress of any kind, including anything that was the slightest threat to peace of mind. In a real sense, these drugs were seen as a scientific triumph and, perhaps, one of the most successful pharmaceutical advances since the Second World War. Yet, when addiction to minor tranquillisers was beginning to become more visible in the mid-1970s, a banner headline, 'A million hooked on instant peace of mind' (*Daily Mail*, 1975) suggested that a medical solution to emotional problems may not be the most beneficial one.

By uncovering some of the 'invisible' issues associated with women's usage of benzodiazepines, the discussions will highlight the intricacies involved in establishing a clear understanding of the women and minor tranquilliser issue. In an attempt to unravel these social complexities, discussions will focus primarily on Britain as a case study.

Maintaining a critical, women-oriented framework helps to challenge misconceptions which are perpetuated in the field. Unless these misconceptions are contested, there is a danger that the field will be insensitive to the needs of many women who are ingesting these 'happiness', 'confidence' and 'peace of mind' pills. There is a need to generate, not inhibit, the development of a feminist perspective in this area of concern.

To develop a feminist analysis a series of interrelated issues will be discussed in this chapter. Firstly, the discussion will look at the workings of the health care 'industry' *vis-à-vis* the pharmaceutical industry and the way that medicine has become a commodity. Identifying women as health care consumers, we then consider how minor tranquillisers maintain passivity as well as stability in the private domestic sphere. Next we look at issues to do with developing an account of the female consumer. The final discussion focuses on developing a women-centred view by identifying how the use of minor tranquillisers can be a way of maintaining an individual's inferiority.

The health care 'industry' and the pharmaceutical industry: medicine as a commodity

The prescription of addictive minor tranquillisers does not occur in a social vacuum. For example, with the evolution of highly sophisticated and technologically based medical systems in developed countries, the health needs of the people using these expensive systems come into conflict with society's requirement for continued capital accumulation. In other words, whether the private sector remains dominant, as in the United States, or whether medical care is organised by the state, as in Britain, this care costs and remains a source of profit.

Reflecting on the origins of the British system of health care as well as writing under the auspices of the ABPI (Association of British Pharmaceutical Industry), Glendenning and Laing (1987, p. 5) clarify this point:

> State provision of medical services was not commonly seen as being a threat to an economic system based upon private ownership, but, on the contrary, was viewed as complementary to it. The welfare state was widely regarded as the social cement that would enhance the prospect of harmony.

In some countries, such as the United Sates and Germany, the rapid expansion of health care costs in recent years have been so unexpected that they have become political issues. That any organised medical system or health care industry cannot operate effectively without its 'curative' drugs, purchased 'privately' from the pharmaceutical industry for vast profits is, however, hidden in the political debates. In Britain, the NHS (National Health Service) is the pharmaceutical industry's principal market, with the proportion of gross output at 45 per cent. Exports rank in second place, comprising 35 per cent of gross output (Association of the British Pharmaceutical Industry, 1986b, p. 6).

With reference to this export market, Doyal (1981, p. 226) has argued that the most important example of 'medicine as a commodity' is provided by the multinational pharmaceutical industry. She notes that, while overall expenditure on medicine in developing countries is much lower than in the developed world, expenditure on drugs is proportionately very much greater. Statistics on UK pharmaceutical exports to developing countries for a ten-year period from 1975 to 1985 reveal a 138 per cent increase, from £73 million to £174 million (Association of the British Pharmaceutical Industry, 1986b, p. 8). In 1986, the industry achieved a record-breaking export performance when overseas sales rose by £100 million to over £1.5 billion, creating a trade surplus in pharmaceuticals of £853 million (Diamond, 1987). Ray (1991, p. 149) suggests that the export of benzodiazepines to developing countries lacks clear regulatory controls and these drugs were often sold in irrational combinations with other drugs or over the counter for trivial conditions. For him, the way these drugs are distributed reflects the global relations of unequal exchange between the developed and developing worlds and contributes to worsening health status in the latter. Let us turn our attention now to a key group of consumers of these drugs.

British women as health care consumers

In 1944, the then Ministry of Health issued a White Paper, *A National Health Service*, on planned objectives for the establishment of a 'state-funded' health service. One of these objectives was:

> to ensure that everyone in the country – irrespective of means, age, sex, or occupation – shall have equal opportunity to benefit from the best and most up-to-date medical and allied services available.

When the NHS was actually established in 1948, it was founded on the belief that a direct investment in health care by the state enhances the nation's prosperity as well as the health of its people. With its development, the principle 'health and well-being as a social right' became established. This right was seen to be financed, administered and indeed safeguarded by the state.

However, in recent years, the main objectives of the NHS have been placed in jeopardy as the result of the introduction of 'free market economy' principles into the debates on its future development. While the NHS has been suffering a number of attacks, it has been shown that there is some connection between the widening social inequalities in health and the widening gap in income between rich and poor (Townsend and Davidson, 1982), that there exists what can be called a 'health divide' in the British health care system (Whitehead, 1987) and that there are clear race, class and gender differences in health and the provision of health services within Britain (Radical Statistics Health Group, 1987).

Since the establishment of the British NHS, women's position as health care consumers has been affected by a variety of social factors. Firstly, there has been a considerable rise in the number of married women in the labour force. In 1951, over 20 per cent of all Britain's married women were employed, as opposed to some 10 per cent in 1931 (Klein, 1965, p. 27). By 1976, it was one in two and, in 1981, two out of three employed women were married (Oakley, 1981). This movement of married women into the labour force has meant that married women who are experiencing the demands of 'domesticity' in the home are also being exposed to the pressures of waged work outside it.

Secondly, it has been shown that social definitions of women have been changing and it is now more socially acceptable to define women as both mothers and workers. Nevertheless Doyal (1981, p. 217) suggests that while definitions of femininity have been liberalised women's essentially domestic and therefore inferior identity ensures their continued oppression and exploitation. In a related context, Sharpe (1984, p. 15) suggests that, while working mothers have a double identity as mothers and workers, society often forgets that married women work because they have to. In effect, the real economic and personal importance of work outside the home tends to be subjugated to the vision of a woman's 'primary' role as wife and mother. What must not be forgotten in this context is that, with the gendered structuring of labour, not only are women less valued as workers than men but also they have access to a more limited range of work (Ramazanoglu, 1989, p. 79).

Thirdly, in recent years the employment of women – both single and married – appears to be moving into decline with the economic recession and rising unemployment levels. During 1979–80, the first two years of the Thatcher government, the annual rate of female unemployment almost doubled, and by the early 1980s unemployment amongst women had increased more than three times faster than that of men (Bruegel, 1982). Overall, between 1976 and 1983, women's unemployment increased fourfold, while men's slightly doubled (Beechey, 1986, p. 102).

During this worsening economic recession women are put into a vulnerable economic position. Women who are employed outside the home are somewhat protected from depression and use few psychotic drugs (Mostow and Newberry, 1975) yet Arber (1990, p. 91) suggests that, for some women, work outside the home may affect their health status if they have little time to do anything except paid work, unpaid domestic labour and routine childcare. Although women need to have a *good health status*, they may be put in a position where they become depressed, become health care consumers and perhaps consume drugs in the face of increasing psychological, physical and emotional stress.

In a classic text, *Social Origins of Depression:A Study of Psychiatric Disorders in Women*, Brown and Harris (1978) demonstrate quite effectively that medical–psychiatric symptoms in women are related to isolation in the home, stress produced by poverty, lack of employment and stressful life events such as bereavement. Furthermore women have a higher incidence of depression than men.

In an apparently compassionate society based on social welfare, public health and individual well-being, people suffering from depression, mental stress, anxiety, or any other symptom which may lead to 'mental illness' tend to be isolated and stigmatised. For women, however, their social position and the nature of their female role as it is constructed are conducive to mental illness. As major health care consumers, women constitute the majority of NHS patients and use the general practitioner, psychiatric, geriatric and most preventative services more frequently than men (Doyal and Elston, 1986, p. 174).

Specifically, in comparison to men, women were found to be one and a half times more likely to enter a psychiatric hospital at some period in their lives (Hill, 1972). Even if we consider the recent fall in psychiatric admissions and the movement to community care over the last 20 years, the difference in the proportions of women and men still remains (Doyal and Elston 1986, p. 175). Women more often than men are categorised as 'depressed', 'psychoneurotic', 'psychotic' or as 'suffering from non-specific disorder' (Lipshitz, 1978). In effect, within a medical framework, women's distress is viewed as a psychiatric disorder alone and more often than not psychotropic drugs are seen as the treatment of choice (Penfold and Walker, 1984, p. 197).

Therefore, as a select group of health care consumers, women are more vulnerable than men to any changes within the health care delivery system. In a broader context, the welfare state is partly concerned with making non-workers, such as unemployed housewives, participate in the economy by consuming the state's services, yet, in recent years, with the growth of private-sector services in Britain, the health care consumer is seen to have more 'choice'. One must be aware that, in the developing economic climate, consumer 'choice' should be understood as meaning increased profits for developing as well as established industries in the private sector. One of these established industries is pharmaceuticals, defined as an 'oligopolistic global organization' (Ray, 1991, p. 149).

The pharmaceutical industry's investment in 'passivity'

One of the most significant and successful penetrations of private capital into the NHS has been through the pharmaceutical industry. Represented by the APBI (Association of British Pharmaceutical Industry), this trade association has over 150 members who provide more than 99 per cent of all medicines supplied through the NHS (ABPI, 1986a).

On a global scale, 20 multinational pharmaceutical companies, such as Merck & Co., Hoechst, Hoffman La Roche, Ciba Geigy, Bayer, American Home Products, ICI and Glaxo accounted for over 51 per cent of worldwide sales in 1985–6. Of these companies, Glaxo and ICI are British, with total pharmaceutical sales for each company amounting to £2.5 billion and £1.5 billion respectively (Parker, 1987). One of the world's largest multinational pharmaceutical companies is Hoechst, based in Frankfurt-am-Main, Germany, with 12 national subsidiaries. Other subsidiaries are based throughout the world in 21 countries. Last year Hoeschst sales amounted to DM 37 billion with a profit of DM 1.5 billion (Hoechst, 1988). The British subsidiary, based in Hounslow, made a profit of £9 million with sales reaching £288 million.

In an ABPI ranking (1986b, p. 10) of the top 12 British industries (excluding the petroleum industry) by size of net foreign exchange earnings, the pharmaceutical industry ranked fourth with earnings valued at £832 million (most recent figures 1985). Perhaps we are beginning to see that public health may have more to do with a healthy pharmaceutical industry than has been previously considered.

It is difficult to establish the exact relationship between the NHS and the pharmaceutical industry. Information produced each year by the Prescription Pricing Authority (PPA) on what drugs are prescribed by the NHS (by brands, quantities and price) is kept confidential by the Department of Health. However we do know that as a proportion of gross NHS cost, expenditure on pharmaceutical services has remained constant at around 10–11 per cent since 1951 (*World Drug Market Manual*, 1986) and that prescription numbers have risen steadily over a period of 40 years since the establishment of the NHS in 1948. For example, in 1949 prescriptions numbered 225.1 million, in 1970 they numbered 306 million, in 1980, 374 million and by 1986 the number was 397 million (Office of Health Economics, 1984; ABPI, 1986b; ABPI, 1987). We also know that in 1977 the NHS drugs bill amounted to £596 million (*Lancet*, 1978), in 1981, £1067.6 million; in 1982 £1233.2 million (Lacey, 1984), in 1984, £1702 million and that by 1986 it was £2031 million (ABPI, 1987).

In 1978, Lader argued that benzodiazepines were the most commonly prescribed type of psychotropic. Recently Williams and Bellantuono (1991) noted that the most frequently prescribed minor tranquillisers in Britain and other industrialised societies are benzodiazepines. Focusing on Britain, Clare (1981) found that psychotropics represented 15 per cent of all prescriptions written by general practitioners (GPs) and 17 per cent of all NHS prescriptions. Williams (1980) pointed out that overall NHS official prescribing statistics for psychotropics do not include drugs prescribed for out-patients and in-patients and therefore must be interpreted cautiously. Furthermore benzodiazepines may be prescribed as tranquillisers, hypnotics or anti-convulsants and these prescriptions may be counted under different drug group headings.

Having developed an interest in this area, the Institute for the Study of Drug Dependence (ISDD, 1987, p. 10) collected information on a variety of local and national surveys on psychotropic drugs. They report:

> One study in 1971 suggested that 12 per cent of the adult population in England and Wales had taken a prescribed psychotropic drug in the previous fortnight and that 7% had first been prescribed that drug a year or more ago . . . A 1984 Mori survey suggested that 23% of the adult population had taken a tranquilliser at some time in their lives and a third of these had taken them for longer than the current recommended limit of 4 months.

With special reference to women they say:

> The proportion of women making short or long term use of prescribed psychotropic drugs is consistently found to be about double the proportion of men, though this sex difference appears to even out among the elderly . . . a third of all women have at some time been

prescribed tranquillisers, over a quarter sleeping pills and . . . very nearly half (46%) of the women in Britain have been prescribed one or other at some time in their life.

In another related report (ISDD, 1989b) they identified:

about 1,250,000 chronic benzodiazepine users in the UK, people who take tranquillisers every day. Of these, two-thirds are women, mostly aged 50 and above. Some have taken tranquillisers for 10 or 20 years.

Before benzodiazepines came onto the market in the 1960s, doctors prescribed amphetamines as daytime anti-depressants, while barbiturates were used for night-time sedation. Some of these drugs became popular on the illicit drug market. By the early 1970s policies were aimed at misusers who obtained these drugs on the 'black market' (Jamieson, Glanz and MacGregor, 1984). In more recent years these drugs have penetrated the illicit market, with resultant abuse by injecting drug users (Black, 1988; Farrell and Strang, 1988; Stimson, Ettorre, Crosier and Stephens, 1991). Doctors themselves set up CURB (Campaign on the Use and Restriction of Barbiturates) in 1975 to help reduce the prescribing of barbiturates. Many switched to prescribing benzodiazepines as a 'safer' alternative.

Changes in prescribing practices suggested that doctors were increasingly prescribing drugs classed as anti-depressants and tranquillisers for night-time sedation. Minor tranquillisers such as benzodiazepines were marketed as being effective as both day-time tranquillisers and night-time sedation. Benzodiazepines were believed to be more effective and safer than barbiturates in alleviating stress and anxiety and in dealing with 'the extent of clinical anxiety in society' (Office of Health Economics, 1982).

Between 1970 and 1975 the number of barbiturate stimulant prescriptions decreased, while for tranquillisers and anti-depressants the number went up (Williams, 1980). This could suggest that while 'barb freaks' were finding it increasingly difficult to get prescriptions to supplement their drug habits, housewives were easily able to obtain tranquillisers to supplement theirs.

As with barbiturates, benzodiazepines have been related to both psychological and physical dependence (Lader, 1983; Marks, 1985; Petursson and Lader, 1986; Golombok, 1991) and the Committee on the Review of Medicines (1980) reported 'the lack of firm evidence of efficacy which might support the long-term use of benzodiazepines in insomnia and anxiety'.

In this context it should be noted that, owing to a variety of factors including increasing public concern about the risks of benzodiazepine dependence, legislation in 1985 limited the range of prescribing of seven categories of drugs under the NHS by setting up an 'acceptable' and 'unacceptable' list of drugs able to be prescribed (Gabe and Williams, 1986). Interestingly enough, those drugs on the 'unacceptable' list could still be obtained privately, which generated a new demand within the private sector. Benzodiazepines have been a major category of drugs on the list (Bury and Gabe, 1990).

In 1986, the regulations under the Misuse of Drugs Act were extended to include benzodiazepines as a Class C, Schedule 4 drug. In effect this meant that, under the Act, it became an offence (that of supplying) for anyone using these drugs on their doctor's prescription to give someone any quantity of their benzodiazepines (ISDD, 1989a), including a single pill.

In the light of the above-mentioned legislative changes, we find that between 1974 and 1985 the total number of benzodiazepine prescriptions rose from 24.6 million in 1974 to a peak of almost 31 million in 1979, falling to 26 million in 1985. While total benzodiazepine prescriptions over the latter six-year period had fallen by 16 per cent, 70 per cent of these drugs were dispensed to women. It was estimated that by the mid-1980s some 13 million British women aged over 40 received almost 60 per cent of all benzodiazepine medicines prescribed for the British population (Taylor, 1987). Heather Ashton and John Golding's (1989) 1985–6 study found that 3 per cent of a random sample of adults in Britain were taking benzodiazepines, suggesting over one million long-term users. Usage was twice as common amongst women and was associated with unemployment, less active leisure pursuits, low socioeconomic status and age.

In 1981, Lader emphasised that the problem of dependence on tranquillisers is particularly relevant to women as they take these drugs and encounter dependence problems twice as frequently as men. Extending this statement, Curran and Golombok (1985, p. 36) argue that tranquillising women is a feminist issue and that only by looking to the circumstances in which women find themselves turning to a bottle of pills can we begin to understand why women run the risk of becoming dependent on drugs.

With nearly 28 million benzodiazepine prescriptions at a cost of over £30 million to the NHS (Shiell, 1991) and given the invisible cost to the lives of thousands of women users, the use of benzodiazepines should be considered a social issue worthy of critical attention. Whether or not we view benzodiazepine use as an 'evil necessity' (Gabe and Lipshitz-Phillips, 1982), as a 'means of social control' (Gabe and Lipshitz-Phillips, 1984), as one of a number of resources available to people to help them cope with modern life (Gabe and Thorogood, 1986a) or as simply a solution to the problems of living (Stimson, 1975b), the issue is about a NHS investment in the image of women as passive consumers. It also concerns the aggressive marketing strategies of the pharmaceutical industry which, like those of the alcohol and diet industries, are aimed at women. For women the result is the perpetuation of their passivity and domesticity.

RELEASE (1982), a national organisation concerned with the problem of tranquillisers and how it relates to women, estimated that the money invested by the pharmaceutical industry in advertising and promotion represents twice the amount spent on research and development. This is a very substantial investment, given that British pharmaceutical research and development costs for 1986 were estimated to be in the order of £550m (Diamond, 1987). Furthermore there is one drug company representative for every eight general practitioners in Britain. Although the pharmaceutical industry talks about 'pharmaco-vigilance' as it develops conditions for access to the European Market (Hankin, 1988), one wonders how 'attentive' the industry will be as regards the needs of women. As the free movement of goods (in this case benzodiazepines) is instituted, along with increased promotion of sales, the 'European woman' may replace the British woman as the advertising target.

Melville (1984) reported that out of 115 drug advertisements for tranquillisers in the *British Medical Journal*, 91 referred directly to women patients. Prather and Fidell (1975) found that advertisements for psychoactive drugs were strongly associated with showing a women as the patient. Geared to women, the message of most psychotropic drug advertisements is that everyday stress, anxiety and depression are medical problems. As a result intervention is oriented towards the individual who is under stress rather than towards a society in need of change (Stimson, 1975a). Women have become a prime market for psychotropic drugs and, during a period of economic recession, society needs to keep its growing number of non-workers (women) in their traditional roles of housewives, mothers, caretakers and nurturers.

In this context, Cooperstock and Lennard (1986) noted that people who experienced problems with their tranquilliser use reported that continued use was seen as a way of permitting them to maintain themselves in roles which they found intolerable without the drugs. For women, the most common roles discussed related to the traditional roles of wife, mother and houseworker. In a similar vein, Estep (1987) points out that women's use of prescribed drugs is very much associated with and influenced by family life.

Developing an account of the female consumer

In the following discussion it is assumed that the development of a social scientific view in the field has facilitated the growth of a critical perspective on benzodiazepines. However, while social scientists have helped to generate an awareness of some of the social aspects of benzodiazepine use, it has been recently argued that the field lacks good sociological research which takes into account the perceptions of the drug's effects as viewed by the 'consumers' and well as the broader political, economic and cultural context of the problem (Gabe, 1990).

More importantly, while research data consistently identify women as primary consumers of psychotropics, and indeed women-oriented perspectives have been put forward (Curran and Golombok, 1985; Melville, 1984; Ettorre, 1985d), the field lacks a theoretical perspective sympathetic to the needs of these female consumers and providing a clear understanding of whether or not women and men use drugs differently.

This lack is not surprising, given that a marriage between a gender-sensitive theoretical approach and sociological research has been problematic (Wallace, 1989) and, specifically, the field of addiction studies has been resistant both theoretically and methodologically to an approach which is sensitive to the needs of women as a social group (Ettorre, 1989b). Research on psychotropic drug use lacks good sociological studies which illuminate the viewpoint of the consumers within a critical women-oriented perspective. Therefore to speak of the development of schools of thought in this area or to identify any major theoretical developments concerning women as primary consumers is a somewhat futile exercise.

The sparse sociological work carried out from a female consumer's viewpoint fails to answer the question as to why for women the use of these addictive substances stems from the particular circumstances in which women find themselves as women. Additionally this type of research unknowingly lends support to a traditional belief that pharmacological aids to relieve anxiety and depression are worthwhile because they have been used throughout history and have more positive than negative individual and social effects (Hallstrom, 1989). This type of research reconfirms established psycho-social findings in the field that there is a clear connection for consumers between the use of psychotropics and stress (Hansen, 1989) and the consumer's need to cope with negative emotions (Craig, Cappell, Busto and Kay, 1987).

This research does not enhance the development of a women-oriented perspective and leaves key questions concerning the 'gender order' unanswered. If a critical women-oriented perspective is to develop, there is a need to investigate how the everyday effects of the 'gender order' are related to the use of psychotropic drugs. Thus far this issue is not explored by sociologists working in the field and this appears as somewhat surprising given that the notion of the gender order has already been established as a crucial sociological factor in analysing health and illness in contemporary society (Stacey, 1988).

While traditional sociological research has been criticised for gender bias (Stanley and Wise, 1983a and b), there is a need for research which emphasises the interplay between the public, primary sphere of social relations and the private, secondary female sphere of social relations. How do these two spheres of social life have an impact on psychotropic drug use – for both men and women? For example, Estep (1987) demonstrates that women's use of prescribed drugs is associated with and influenced by family life. Does family life in some way influence men's use of psychotropics and if so, in what ways?

Furthermore, there is a need to look at attitudes about the use of psychotropic drugs outside traditional treatment settings? Users already being processed in the treatment system or those already seeking help are the subjects of sociological research in this area and this may distort the image of the consumer. What about individuals who experience stress, who may have used these drugs but who seek alternatives? Self-help groups can be a viable alternative to psychotropic drug use (Ettorre, 1986b), what about other alternatives such as counselling programmes (Shiell, 1991)? Are certain sub-groups of men (such as unemployed men, 'house husbands', lorry drivers, teachers and sportsmen) using psychotropics more than other sub-groups of men and, if so, why?

Let us now focus specifically on the unique social position of the woman tranquilliser user and begin to develop a feminist account. Emphasising the reasons for a women-oriented perspective in this area, Morell (1981, p. 38) discusses how the need to prevent more of what she calls 'prescription drug dependence of women' must be linked with a conscious feminist stance. She suggests that, if our work is not intentionally feminist, it 'leads to victim blaming and encourages individual women to absorb responsibility for more than their share of what are in fact social problems'.

The reasons why women use psychotropic drugs are similar to the reasons why women get depressed (Nairne and Smith, 1984), Both psychotropic drug use and depression can be seen as an escape from the oppressive nature of the domestic role – a role located in the private sphere, the home. In structurally powerless positions of wife and patient in relation to husband and doctor (Barrett and Roberts, 1978) a woman is trained to gain whatever comforts, joys or pleasures she can. The supply of psychotropics is allowed by the state, promoted by the pharmaceutical industry and 'demanded' by the female patient who asks, 'Doctor, will you give me something to make me feel better, less anxious, less stressed and less depressed?' The hidden question is, 'Doctor, can you help me to feel less socially inferior?' Often the answer to both questions is a minor tranquilliser.

The relationship between women and the medical profession, particularly psychiatry (Showalter, 1985) can be seen historically as a relationship of social control (Ehrenreich and English, 1974) and the medical belief in the inferiority of women is clearly reflected in the widespread assumption that most women are 'neurotic' (Doyal,

1981). The consequences of this relationship and this belief is that women more than men become dependent on the institution of medicine for help.

The relationship any woman who uses tranquillisers may have to her doctor may reveal a collusion process in which denial of feelings is paramount. By prescribing drugs, the most a doctor can hope for is that the symptoms of anxiety or depression will be alleviated for a while (Curran and Golombok, 1985, p. 40). By accepting this process, a woman may be denied as well as deny an active role in maintaining her supply of 'her drug'. Tranquillisers do not solve the underlying problem or problems a woman may be experiencing and may create further problems (Women's National Commission, 1988, p. 71).

On the other hand, long-term consumption of 'her drug' may be consistent with her own social-cum-psychological expectation to 'be a good girl' (that is, to be dependent) and 'to follow her doctor's orders' (doctor knows best). Yet minor tranquillisers will change neither society's expectation of her as a 'dependent' woman nor her husband, job, children and all the rest. If the woman tranquilliser user emerges from the private sphere she is less of a threat to the established order. As both 'strung-out patient' and 'dutiful wife', she may remain less visible than her heroin-using counterpart: the female junkie. As implied in an earlier discussion, the woman tranquilliser user is managed and manageable in an environment legitimated by male authority: her husband's and her doctor's. In a real sense she enacts a rejection of what could be termed the 'super-mum' syndrome in this structurally powerless position. In this private sphere, tranquilliser use may be, whether consciously or not, a housewife's only recourse to comfort and relief from stress and, regardless of the initial reason or reasons for a woman actively consuming tranquillisers, she perpetuates the image of women as 'passive consumers'.

Unlike a woman heroin user, she affirms the social image of women as dependent. On the one hand she is, similar to most women an active health care consumer *vis-à-vis* her tranquilliser prescription. On the other hand, her passive consumption of tranquillisers in the domestic sphere confirms and epitomises her dependency, of both the 'addiction' and 'subordinate thing' kind. As a passive consumer she is not, however, a passive victim. In the fullest sense, she is a dependent woman more than a 'non-woman'. While she may consciously choose to 'pollute' her body (her internal environment) with 'mind-altering substances' (her tranquillisers), her dependent position does not allow her to transgress the boundaries of this dependency in order to pollute the public sphere. Unlike the woman heroin user (Perry, 1979), the femininity of the woman tranquilliser user is not 'misplaced', 'defied' and 'defiled'. Her femininity remains intact as she is relatively 'well placed', contained/containable, managed/manageable under the auspices of the family. While her daily 'tranx fix' helps her to cope with the monotonous grind and to dampen feelings of self-worth, she remains in the eyes of society unfeminine, sexless, devalued as a woman and deskilled as the primary psychological coper in the family.

Regardless of where women's substance use may be located (in the public or the private sphere), all women substance misusers emerge as insufficiently feminine, uncaring about men and risking the loss of their attention and approval. Within the context of what Sterling (1989) terms the 'tranquillising of society', dependence on tranquillisers may induce a sense of guilt and shame for some women tranquilliser users. In this atmosphere the pharmaceutical industry's response has been to promote more socially fashionable products, such as vitamins which have higher consumer acceptability. Let us now focus our attention on the way a women-centred view can be developed.

Developing a women centred view

In an article on the long-term use of tranquillisers, Helman (1986) examines the symbolic role that these particular drugs play in the lives of long-term users and classifies three main groups: tonic, fuel and food. The respective groups' gender composition was 71 per cent, 78 per cent and 100 per cent female. While each grouping represents a different conceptualisation or symbolic meaning of psychotropic drugs and their use, they are not discrete groups, but rather clusters of attributes. Helman's classification has important implications for the development of a woman-centred perspective in this area. Simply, his work demonstrates quite clearly how any woman's use of an 'acceptable' prescribed drug masks their invisible *desire* to be an 'acceptable' woman in society. For example, taking a tonic evidences the need to control one's life, taking fuel evidences the need to function 'normally' and lastly, taking food evidences the need to survive. Regardless of the hidden desires of woman tranquilliser users, their 'doctor's love affair with benzodiazepines' (Mondanaro, 1989, p. 110) makes them into neurotic females as well as drugging them into a state where they cannot achieve their desire to be an acceptable, non-neurotic female. As one woman (an ex-tranquilliser user) explains:

> The word 'tranquilliser' has particularly nasty connotations for me, because I was once in a state of nervous depression while I was a student . . . I knew what it was like to be in a nervous depression and I knew it wasn't what was wrong with me now. But he was bringing it all back, with all his glib assumptions and easy answers, which left me totally out of account. He was creating in me the very thing on which doctors blame so many wasted surgery hours: the neurotic female . . . And there you have it. Woman seen through the eyes of man, treated with the male as a reference point, even when diagnosed (wrongly) as having a traditional female complaint. (Bardsley, 1984, p. 208)

Women tranquilliser users have emerged in a traditional role, as 'passive consumer', through the ignorance and insensitivity of some members of the medical profession. This process has contributed to feelings of inferiority. Until women become conscious of their need for pleasure and more importantly their need for pleasure without drugs, their role as passive consumers may be perpetuated. Furthermore, unless women begin to recognise their potential for integrity, dignity and self-respect as women, there will be no remedy for their forced alienation from themselves.

For Dworkin (1987, p. 169), this forced alienation is the essence of women's 'inferiority'.

> Inferiority is the deep and destructive devaluing of a person in life, a shredding of dignity and self-respect, an imposed exile from human worth and human recognition, the forced alienation of a person from even the possibility of wholeness or internal integrity. Inferiority puts rightful self-love beyond reach, a dream fragmented by insult into a perpetually recurring nightmare; inferiority creates a person broken and humiliated inside. The fragments – scattered pieces and sharp slivers of someone who can never be made whole – are then taken to be the standard of what is normal in her kind: women are like that.

In a powerful and vivid account of her painful experiences as a minor tranquilliser user, Barbara Gordon (1979, p. 51) refers to her drug (Valium) as 'a leveller'. She says, 'It evens things out silently, quietly. No rush, no thrill, no charge . . . the safe and sane drug.' Any woman tranquilliser user may experience the need to 'even things out silently'. From a feminist perspective, this need can be translated into the need to stay 'inferior' while feeling inferior. In other words, the user hears the cultural injunction: 'Be like a woman: second-class, needy, neurotic and naturally dependent.' While these drugs may help her to 'stop making a fuss' about the contradictory feelings she is feeling as a woman, she is levelled out, unable to fight back and separated off from any positive form of resistance. Rather than being empowered she is 'depowered'.

In this context women may need to take risks or become adventurous. Whether or not they share Vance's (1984, p. 24) view that 'it is not safe to be a woman', they need to explore carefully somewhat 'dangerous' notions such as becoming an active consumer – taking control of one's drug use or claiming and searching for pleasure. These notions, if acted upon, would challenge their current situation.

On the hierarchy of addictions, tranquillisers are seen as good, safe and socially necessary to maintain stability and sanity in the private sphere. While the widespread use of benzodiazepines may be visible as a 'mass cultural phenomenon' (Bellantuono *et al.*, 1980), the pharmaceutical industry's massive profits in the public sphere tend to remain invisible. While women, the passive consumers, are consistently caught up in this social quagmire, they appear to be the primary consumers whose desires, needs and pleasures remain invisible. In effect doctors' prescriptions, along with society's prescription that women are to be dependent, shadow the valid experiences that women, whether as individuals or a collective, have as independent, self-loving and powerful human beings.

In conclusion, it could be argued that women's use of minor tranquillisers is a 'dismembering process' in which women's minds are cut of from their bodies, their feelings from reality and their emotions from pleasure. To right this process women users, whatever their social, class or racial position, need to Re-member or simply, to 'Re-call the Original intuition of integrity and to heal the dismembered self' (Daly, 1988, p. 92).

To effect lasting changes women users need to examine how their sense of integrity is more often than not entwined with an ethic of care based on helping and pleasing others rather than themselves.

Women minor tranquilliser users need to move themselves away from the ethic of care to the ethic of responsibility. While recognising the gendered nature of caring, women users need to create mechanisms for the preservation of their own sense of integrity. Whatever the chosen options, women need to move away from seeing themselves as flawed or inferior. As Gilligan (1982, pp. 171–2) rightly states:

> When the distinction between helping and pleasing frees the activity of taking care from the wish for approval by others, the ethic of responsibility can become a self-chosen anchor of personal integrity and of strength . . . Rather than viewing her anatomy as destined to leave her with a scar of inferiority, one can see instead how it gives rise to experiences which illuminate a reality common to both of the sexes: the fact that in life you never see it all, that things unseen undergo change through time, that there is more than one path to gratification and that boundaries between self and other are less clear than they sometimes seem.

As women benzodiazepine users move away from the ethic of care to the ethic of responsibility, they learn to heal their dismembered selves. On a deep level, they learn more to Re-member and to find their own women-centred, self-chosen anchors based on a sense of personal integrity and inner strength.

4

Women and heroin

A 'Horror' story, sold as the typical female 'addict': Tiny Jodie Carroll knew no cause for the torments she experienced at her birth – but her mother, Kathy did. Because of 17-year-old Kathy's heroin habit, her baby was born an addict. 'Even when I was pregnant I couldn't go without a fix', she said. (*Women's Own*, 'Heroin: the peddlers of death' 28 January 1984)

Introduction

Unlike other chapters in this book, this chapter will examine illicit drug use, specifically the use of an illegal substance, heroin. Similar to other chapters, it is based on discussions and analyses informed by feminist theory. Most work on women heroin users focuses on the official drug treatment system. This chapter looks both within and beyond the official drug treatment system. A main assumption here is that women addicts, similar to women alcoholics within the official treatment system, have been treated in ways that have stifled their empowerment and their growth as women. There is a need to look beyond the drug treatment system to the women themselves in order to have a clear idea of the problems they face. The dynamics of their unique social positioning as 'deviant women' will be challenged.

Discussions in this chapter will also attempt to break down the misconceptions about women's use of heroin. From the standpoint of the 'hierarchy of drugs', we look objectively at the way women's use of heroin is viewed as bad and morally reprehensible.

The main topics presented in this chapter include discussions about how heroin can be seen as a masculine drug and the ramifications for women users; why female heroin users are perceived as polluted women; heroin use as 'spoiling one's identity as a women; women heroin users' experience of the drug treatment system and women, prostitution, injecting drug use and HIV/AIDS. All of these discussions should provide the reader with a direct insight into the existing state of affairs within the field.

Heroin: a 'masculine' drug?

In any discussion on heroin it is useful to know that the word comes from the German word 'heroisch', meaning heroic or mighty (Whitaker, 1987). Reflecting on the etymological roots of this word may lead one to consider that heroin is perceived more as a male drug than a female drug. Simply, keeping the root meaning of the word 'heroin' in mind, one considers that generally men more than women are thought to be 'mighty' or 'heroic'. On the other hand, in a search for a female equivalent to the male 'mighty', one finds images such as Joan of Arc or the Amazons as mighty or heroic women. However these images are somewhat flawed: Joan of Arc was considered to be a witch and the Amazons were viewed as single-breasted perverts. If then heroin is the 'king' of drugs, one wonders why women drug users ever got involved. The story is not a simple one.

For example, any picture of the prevalence of female heroin use is clouded by the fact that there is no way of determining the total number of women dependent upon heroin. Examinations of official statistics and survey reports are not very useful in providing a picture of the prevalence of female heroin use because they tend to represent a minority of users (that is, those users of notifiable drugs seeking help) or a select treatment population. In Britain, it appears that a third of the drug-using population are women. According to Home Office statistics, there were a total of 4306 female users of notifiable drugs in 1989, accounting for 29 per cent of the total number of notifications (Home Office, 1990) In 1990, there was a slight increase in the number of female users (4948), but these women accounted for a slightly lower percentage (28 per cent) of the total number (Home Office, 1991).

In the United States opiate use has been increasing among women at a greater rate than among men. A look at selected treatment populations in the 1970s reveals that women represented about 30 per cent of the total client population in heroin treatment programmes, while in earlier years it was estimated to be around 18 per cent (Hser, Anglin and McGlothin, 1987). However Glover Reed (1987) points out that during the late 1980s the large majority of treatment programmes continued with a 2:1 to 10:1 imbalance of men to women. Whatever indicators of women's drug use exist, it is clear that this information is of limited use in providing a comprehensive picture of women's use of heroin.

Yet it appears that the current explanations of women's use of heroin offered by society's 'experts' are all that is needed to understand this problem. These explanations, with few exceptions, tend to uphold traditional images of women as weak, passive, dependent and responsible for caring for others physically, psychologically and emotionally. The drug-using world, although separated in our minds from mainstream culture, emerges from within a society that perpetuates a powerful anti-drug ideology. For example, governments talk about a 'War on Drugs' and politicians refer to the 'evils of drug use'. Nevertheless this illicit drug-using world reflects similar dynamics of oppression institutionalised in wider society. The politics of gender, race and class operate to keep minority groups from having much access (if any) to political power. Clearly these dynamics operate in the drug-using world.

In society's eyes, women as members of the illicit drug-using world of heroin have failed as women. As failures, they have abandoned their role as guardians of moral standards. Ryle (1987) argues that the growth of uncontrollable drug use may be a symptom of the moral disorganisation of society as well as a refuge from it. Within this view, women heroin users are appropriately victimised as one of the major perpetrators of the moral breakdown of society.

In this context Rosenbaum (1981) in her study of women heroin users found that more than twice as many women as men became dependent on heroin after initial use. Furthermore women proceeded more swiftly to regular daily use than men. For many of these women daily use depended on availability. Not surprisingly, most of these women were living with men who were drug dealers. Other researchers (Hser, Anglin and McGlothin, 1987) maintain that the initial use of heroin by a woman is highly influenced by a man, especially a sex partner, who is often a daily heroin user.

With women-sensitive eyes, Rosenbaum notes that a heroin-using woman, like her non-drug-using female counterpart, is expected to bond with a man and share, indeed support, many aspects of his life. For the female partner of a male heroin user her role is clear: she should share this activity, albeit an illicit one, with her man. On the one hand, she thereby abandons her moral stewardship; on the other, she upholds traditional sex role stereotypes by identifying with her male partner and by upholding social expectations that she share with him his important life activities.

From a very different perspective, other drug researchers (Chein, Gerard, Lee and Rosenfeld, 1964) have argued that women heroin users deny their passive natures by using drugs. Given that it has also been argued that women's use of illicit drugs is an indication of a recent trend towards social equality for women, this is an interesting observation. For example, some women are seen to be adopting independent if not rebellious life styles that include the recreational use of illicit drugs, such as heroin (Suffet and Brotman, 1976). In order to fit adequately into these models of explanation, women need to appear as more assertive than is generally expected. As discussed above, the traditional expectation is that the woman heroin user is relatively passive and dependent upon her man. However, regardless of whether or not women are seen to be passive or aggressive in their use of drugs, women heroin users are clearly subjected to the same social expectations and forms of subordination as many women in society.

While the above discussion presents various explanations for women's use of heroin, it is perhaps illuminating to focus on a specific image of the female heroin user: the polluted woman. A clear perspective on the complex structural dynamics confronting women drug users will be put forward. Also the subtle ways in which women more than men drug users encounter oppressive and sometimes subtle patriarchal practices will be outlined.

Female heroin users as 'polluted' women

Women who use heroin are seen to be polluted women. To develop an understanding of this notion one needs to look at the way two related notions, internal pollution and pollution, have been traditionally defined in the social scientific community. The Introduction to this book alluded to a current definition of 'internal pollution' as 'the state when the purity of the internal environment of our bodies is destroyed' (Warburton, 1978) and the extension of this argument was shown to be victim blaming. More importantly, if links with this previous discussion are made with ideas presented here, women heroin users seen to experience internal pollution become prime targets in this victimisation process. In the light of these ideas, the following discussion of the general notion of pollution should clarify why it is that women more than men heroin users are designated within the victim role.

Mary Douglas has defined pollution as 'a type of danger which is unlikely to occur except where the lines of structure cosmic or social are clearly defined' (Douglas, 1966, p. 113). She suggests that in the light of women's social position, social boundaries created by these lines of structure are more clearly defined for women than for men. Given the above, it could be argued that the consequence of transgressing these social boundaries (poisoning themselves, being out of control and so on) for women heroin users is stigmatisation and/or ostracism. In a real sense these women have polluted or spoiled identities. For example, in private they are viewed as potentially sexless, bad mothers, uncaring for their children or irresponsible wives, not considering the needs of their husbands. In public they are viewed as unforgivably out of control in their domestic and/or work situations, fallen angels, evil sluts or loose women who cannot be trusted and should be avoided. In a related context, Nurco, Wegner and Stephensen (1982, p. 78) emphasise the low, irrevocable status of the female drug addict. They contend that she is seen as 'trash, degraded, the lowest form of life, dope fiend, bum, bitch, stinking whore, despicable, dirty and they will do anything for a shot'.

Feminist scholars have suggested that women have an unenviable role as bearers of uncontrollable emotions (that is, those aspects of human experience which we least understand or have the least control over) (Miller, 1978; Ernst and Goodison, 1981). Additionally, in the private/female sphere of domestic life, women, particularly mothers, have been shown to be the primary emotional copers, with potential risk to their physical and mental well-being (Graham, 1983, 1984; Brown and Harris, 1978). These social roles and resultant practices have particular ramifications for women heroin users. Regardless of when, where, how and why they take heroin, such women are thought to have polluted their bodies and their identities as women. In turn they have 'spoiled' the private sphere of 'domestic bliss' and the public sphere of social hygiene. In effect, women heroin users are polluted women *par excellence.*

For any woman the social expectation that she will behave in traditional – that is, dependent – ways is clear. Nevertheless an incompatibility exists between the social expectation for women to be dependent and the need for all women to be 'in control'. For example, a woman, any woman, by being dependent on a male-oriented structure, such as the family, can be viewed as being controlled by a man (whether consciously or not). By being controlled, she is seen to be in control of her life. A woman heroin user may consciously choose to use a dependent substance in order to cope with or to be in control of an oppressive, controlling situation such as family life. Regardless of how she sees herself, she is viewed as a woman out of control and not a normal woman. The real, underlying message for a woman is that, at all times, she should be in control of herself, mindful of her spouse, her children, her domestic responsibilities and her work situation. If she feels strung out, stressed, unable to cope, she should avoid mind-altering substances. As we have seen in the previous chapter, there are exceptions. The use of tranquillisers can usually be managed or contained in the 'controlled' environment of the home through the authority of the husband and/or the prescribing doctor, who are usually male.

Recalling the hierarchy of drugs discussed earlier, we see that there are drugs ranging from 'good or more socially acceptable drugs' such as alcohol and tranquillisers at the top of the hierarchy and 'bad or unacceptable drugs' such as cocaine and heroin at the bottom. This hierarchy, dependent on our social value system and primitive notions of pollution and purity, obviously affects both men and women substance users. However the social demarcation of the public and private spheres places women more than men in a socially vulnerable position if they choose to consume mind-altering substances, particularly an illicit drug such as heroin.

Female heroin use: 'spoiling' one's identity

A close examination of the images and social practices of women heroin users in the two distinct spheres of social life, the public and the private, reveals how heroin use challenges traditional female stereotypes and roles related to the identity of a 'real' woman. For example, as Perry (1979, p. 3) demonstrates quite eloquently, the female 'junkie' or 'pusher' in the public sphere represents femininity misplaced, defied and defiled. Specifically the female 'junkie' and/or 'pusher' is the embodiment of a woman who *rejects* her femininity. In the public sphere, she is a 'non-woman'. Her visibility is a direct challenge to the established, patriarchal order. Additionally, if she is a prostitute, as are some female 'junkies', she characterises a woman who is doubly polluted because she consumes drugs on the illegal market and 'produces' illicit sex consumed by male clients. However whether or not a woman heroin user is a prostitute is perhaps not that significant. This is mainly because a female 'junkie' is seen as prostituting her identity. Whether or not a female heroin addict has ever exchanged her body for drugs or money for her habit, she is characterised as an impure woman, an evil slut or a loose female. (This link between prostitution and heroin use will be pursued further in the final section of this chapter.)

Regardless of where women's heroin use can be located (in the public or the private sphere), female addicts emerge as insufficiently feminine, uncaring about men and risking the loss of male attention and approval. As Brownmiller (1984, p. 3) suggests, 'to be insufficiently feminine is viewed as a failure in core sexual identity, or as a failure to care sufficiently about oneself, for a woman found wanting will be appraised as mannish or neutered or simply unattractive, as men have defined these terms.' In effect any 'polluted woman' is seen to reject her identity as a woman. She spoils her identity.

Yet it is clear that some women married to heroin-using husbands and coping with children and household chores are upholding their particular gender identities. For example, in traditional working-class families, women tend to see to the child rearing and household chores. Drug addiction does not necessarily alter the structural position of these women, as they look forward to poverty, loss of their good looks, middle age and frustration.

Tam Stewart (1987, p. 106) illustrates quite clearly the effects of this type of situation on women heroin users. She says:

> I have seen female addicts scurry about the house struggling to keep going while their men sprawled about in peaceful drugged slumber like

sated lions on a hot afternoon . . . A woman with a home to run can become very exhausted yet the man often sits by and lets her get on with it. He has his own problems and retreats behind drugs. The man often looks five years younger than he really is and the woman ten years older.

Women in the above situation may need to do the 'scoring' (buying the drugs) for their husbands. Some of these women may resort to shoplifting as a way to obtain money for these drugs. In another context, a 29-year-old married mother and heroin addict (since the age of 13) describes her life before she sought treatment:

We used to nick TVs from Harrods. When you're doing £100 of smack a day, you can't be a secretary. You have to be brazen. I'd carry my goods out of the main entrance and get a porter to call a taxi for me. When you're desperate you take chances . . . If it wasn't TVs it would be silk blouses costing £200 each. They'd go for £90 on the street. (quoted in Laurance, 1987, p. 10)

Some women in such situations may feel that they have become 'neutered' as women. Indeed they may see themselves as not having independent value and status as women. While their heroin use may be intrinsically involved with their relationship with their man, these women, along with others, may view themselves as being less of a woman. For other women addicts, there may be times when they will be driven to prostitute themselves to obtain money to buy drugs for themselves and their husbands.

Aware that she is describing an 'ideal type' of a woman heroin user (that is, on 'one end of a continuum'), Metherell (undated) offers quite a different picture of women heroin users, particularly those who have been driven to exchange sex for drugs when short of cash:

To survive and maintain her habit, she needs to be tough, aggressive, cold, hard, manipulative and tough and she acts that way . . . when she prostitutes herself, she may offer herself and take the money without delivering the goods – in some ways a more risky undertaking. Her body, her sexuality are instruments she uses for gain and for power and dominance. For while some may see her as the victim, as being used, in her own eyes, in her own mind she is in control – the guy is the sucker. She is using him. Her own feelings are not involved. They are satisfied through the drugs she will buy.

Referring specifically to the bond between a woman addict and her partner, Metherell goes on to say:

> She is the strong partner, keeping the home together, earning the money. Without her, her man goes to pieces, cannot cope with life. She is an outsider, strong and independent. What are society's values to her? A hypocritical trap!

It is interesting to note that in all of the above descriptions, the women are in control and apparently caring for their men and their children, rather than out of control and uncaring of others – images which tend to be thrust upon women heroin users by society. While these women may appear as having polluted or spoiled female identities, they are nonetheless women carers with domestic responsibilities for men and children. Regardless of the public images foisted upon them by society, it is clear that these women exert a certain level of control within their private spheres of activity.

Related to these ideas, Jeffries' (1983) argument is that heroin is an aid in helping women to conform to a way of life which is becoming increasingly intolerable. This way of life is intolerable because of its 'unnatural forced values and expectations, especially for those labelled wife and mother'. In the light of these comments, women heroin users are seen to struggle on to keep the family together. Without heroin they are unable to continue to function. On a different note, what happens to these women addicts when they seek help from caring agencies? This is the topic of the next discussion.

Women and the drug treatment system

For many women heroin users, facing treatment and asking for help is a very important step in their lives. A woman heroin user may be overcome by insecurity and fear, particularly if she has a child or children. Given these emotional factors, it is essential that the drug treatment system should be welcoming. Yet the ability of drug treatment agencies to attract women is questionable and little progress has been made in providing what Glover Reed (1987) refers to as 'gender-sensitive services'.

Similar to their alcohol-using counterparts, women heroin users will inevitably find discrimination. (See Chapter 2 for a full discussion of the issue of treatment for women problem drinkers.) Unlike the case of a woman problem drinker, the woman heroin user's substance use is illegal. It could be argued that the illegality of her drug use tends to create a more precarious and chaotic life style than if she were an alcohol abuser. Therefore asking for help becomes a positive step towards living a more stable life, avoiding either arrest or imprisonment. However, given the inadequacy of the drug treatment system and the high relapse rate for women, one may rightly ask 'Is there life after drug use for women'? (Murphy and Rosenbaum, 1987).

Research literature reveals that the majority of both male and female addicts are initiated into drug use by a man (Hser, Anglin and McGlothlin, 1987). As we saw in the above discussion, women who begin daily use of heroin do so mainly because it is easily available – they are living with a male dealer or user who induces them to use 'smack'. While it is unusual for a male heroin user to report having wanted to try drugs because his partner (wife or girlfriend) used them, it is common for women users to be introduced to drugs by their male partners. Women tend to speak of a 'male friend' who exerts pressure on them to use it (Nurco, Wegner and Stephensen, 1982). Additionally Cuskey (1982) found that most first-time women heroin users did not purchase their initial doses of heroin but were offered the drug by men.

One gets the picture that, within the world of illegal use of drugs, specifically heroin, both distribution networks and dealing structures are actively controlled by men (Erickson and Watson, 1990). Not surprisingly, the world of drug treatment is also controlled by men (Brownlee, 1981) and women seeking help in this system tend to find treatment strategies (counselling, psychotherapy, group therapy and so on) sexist in content as well as in form. One study of females in treatment (Soler, Ponsor and Abod, 1976) found that half of the women in their study had been propositioned by male staff members. Refusal to comply with these advances often meant some form of reprisal. This type of behaviour on the part of the male treaters can hardly be seen to be helpful to women drug users, their therapeutic progress or their ultimate recovery. Seeking help and being treated should lessen rather than exacerbate a crisis. One author (Soler, 1980) suggests that women with drug problems are more readily identified and treated within programmes designed specifically to treat women in crisis. The element of crisis for women in treatment tends to remain unrecognised in drug treatment agencies.

Furthermore, within established drug treatment settings, women are particularly vulnerable to the application of a disease model. As Marsh (1982, p. 155) aptly states, 'the disease model fosters a dependency that is counterproductive to treatment; can be used as a basis for coercion; provides too much power to the profession and diverts attention from social and economic influences on drug use'. In this way, medical solutions are often provided to the exclusion of other important service needs for women (such as housing, employment or legal assistance).

For instance, what about the needs of the pregnant woman who is also a drug user? Do these women avoid normal antenatal care for fear of having their newborn baby taken away from them or put on the 'at risk' list? In December 1986 the Law Lords in Britain dismissed an appeal from the guardian of a baby taken into care by Berkshire County Council's social services because the mother was a heroin user during pregnancy. This type of ruling bolsters the prejudicial views held about women illegal drug users: they are unfit to be mothers. As regards this particular case, Perry (1987) says: 'any parent using illegal drugs or having used them during pregnancy faces the dangers of losing custody of their children no matter what the circumstances of the case'. Dixon (1987, p. 6) contends that health service professionals need to provide care for these women in order to help them cope with pregnancy and the long term care of their children.

One health worker outlined a 'non-threatening package' to help pregnant drug users present early enough for good antenatal care (Kearney, 1987). This package would include factors such as HIV pre-test and post-test counselling, the possibility of termination and counselling as well as liaison with other appropriate professionals. Objectively, regardless of whether or not a pregnant woman uses drugs, she should be the one to decide upon the termination or continuation of her pregnancy. The decision should not be in the hands of her treaters or social services.

In this context, a well-known British GP involved in the drug treatment system noted that he had been impressed by the therapeutic effects that child bearing may have on the woman drug user (Women's National Commission, 1988, p. 91). The implication here is that pregnancy is seen as a major incentive to change one's life and give up drugs. If this type of argument is used, there is a danger that women drug users could be propelled into child bearing and child rearing in an uncritical way. In other words, a woman needs to be aware of the realities of motherhood and the fact that for some women (especially those living in poverty) being a mother may be as stressful or more stressful than living the life of a chaotic heroin user. Here the implication is that those involved in the treatment and care of women heroin users need to ensure that the reproductive rights of the women they treat are upheld.

Treatment services also need to account for drug-using mothers who will be especially vulnerable to feeling guilty and blaming themselves for everything (Zuckerman, Amaro and Beardslee, 1987). In their report, *Stress and Addiction amongst Women*, the Women's National Commission (1988) noted that there are too few mother and baby units for the treatment and rehabilitation of women heroin users in Britain. The paucity of special services for these women should not be surprising in the light of society's attitudes towards drug users, which are more censorious for women than for men drug users. While the needs of women heroin users appear to be distinct from those of their male companions, the special needs of mothers and their children should be supported and expanded (Rosenbaum and Murphy, 1987).

Litt (1981) in a study of drug use among adolescent females contends that their drug use has serious social, psychological, physical and medical implications which are both qualitatively as well as quantitatively different from those of adult males in general and male adolescents in particular. Emphasising a clear qualitative difference between adult male and female drug users, Tucker (1982) demonstrates that the pattern of coping by using drugs differed between women and men: simply, women more than men tended to use drugs when they lacked social supports. Treatment settings therefore need to address these gender differences and, more importantly, the disparity between attitudes towards male and female drug users. In this context Colton (1981) asserts that treatment settings must confront these areas of concern or be in danger of 'shirking their responsibility to their female clients'.

Given the complexities of the issues cited in the above discussion, it seems that the option of women-only treatment settings could be considered as a valid one for women heroin users. Marsh (1982) argues that 'an all female treatment modality is a far superior treatment approach to a mixed-sex modality'. In another context, the same author (Marsh, 1981), reporting findings from an all-female programme in Detroit, states that this type of programme provides 'a treatment option that is of value for seriously addicted women and it is imperative that this option be provided'. A woman-only facility explores the idea that many concerns of drug-using women are not dealt with adequately in mixed-sex settings. As has been demonstrated by other authors (Mandel, Schulman and Monteiro, 1979), women focused concerns are important aspects for the rehabilitation and growth of women drug users.

Finally the needs of women drug users who are black (Mauge, 1981; McCarthy and Hirschel, 1984; Kail and Lukoff, 1984a, 1984b); lesbians (Madl, 1981; Miller, 1981; Finnegen and McNally, 1987); medical professionals (Roth, 1987); in the military (Laban, Bell, Vernon and Purcell, 1981) and incarcerated (Miner and Gurta, 1987) should be considered in any comprehensive treatment response. These 'special' groups of women need to find positive ways forward in order to survive in unsupportive environments and social settings. In particular there is a need to ensure that treatment options work against institutionalised racism and homophobia, which are often evident in helping agencies.

No contemporary exploration of the area of women and heroin use would be complete without a discussion of the impact of AIDS (Acquired Immune Deficiency Syndrome) on the female drug-using community. On a worldwide scale, of the eight to ten million adults infected with the virus, more than three million are women. The final section of this chapter will now address this issue.

Women, prostitution, injecting drug use and HIV/AIDS

Currently prostitutes and injecting drug users are being blamed for transmitting AIDS to the heterosexual community. Significantly, traditional myths and images of female drug users are being revitalised in an attempt to obscure the links between sex, gender and power in this emerging field of interest (Butt, 1989). An understanding of these key issues is necessary for a full understanding of the impact of AIDS/HIV infection within the female drug-using population, but a full understanding of these issues tends to be lost in the debates. For example, Wodak (1986) notes:

> As AIDS spreads throughout IV drug users by practice of needle sharing and sexual contacts, female intravenous drug users will increasingly become seropositive. As this group largely generates income to pay for their habit by engaging in prostitution the potential for more rapid transmission of the epidemic through the general community is apparent.

There are some difficulties with this and similar statements which are being expressed in the current AIDS debate. Firstly, an assumption is made that female drug users will usually engage in prostitution to support their habit. A second and somewhat hidden assumption is that, if a woman is a prostitute, she will automatically transmit the virus sexually. In other words, she will not practise safer sex with her male customers. Thirdly, drug-using prostitutes are seen to be in some way removed from the general community, regardless of the fact that the majority of their customers are males, the primary social actors in this community with its white, heterosexual and middle-class bias.

In this context Padian (1988) calls for vigilance in making generalisations about the role that prostitutes play in HIV transmission. She argues that there are cultural differences in the prevalence of and acceptability of prostitution and that research reporting may represent real trends or real trends may be masked by a reporting bias. Prostitutes may be at a higher risk of being infected by their customers than vice versa, since it appears that the efficiency of female to male transmission is lower than male to female transmission. Padian then argues that prostitutes comprise a heterogeneous group and generalisations may depend upon which group of prostitutes are being studied.

While it is important to keep the issues of safer sex and risk-reduction models of treatment (the provision for clean injecting equipment for injecting drug users) in the forefront of discussions on HIV/AIDS-prevention strategies (Stimson, 1989; Richardson, 1987; DAWN, 1988a), there is a need to be sensitive to the fact that women, as James (1987) suggests, 'are being both ignored and scapegoated at the same time'.

For example, major health education campaigns have been directed at both heterosexual and homosexual men, encouraging them to use condoms during penetrative sex, yet, in a very subtle way, women are given the major responsibility for the prevention of the spread of AIDS in the heterosexual community. As Henderson (1990, p. 14) suggests: 'Much of the public health education on HIV/AIDS geared to heterosexuals has placed the responsibility for promoting safer sex, as birth control, upon women.'

In this context, it is not surprising that in some major cities and rural areas throughout both the developed and developing world, prostitutes are being singled out and indeed used as safer sex educators. Whether or not women are prostitutes, they have been traditionally responsible for contraception, therefore it is more than likely that the burden will remain on them to ensure that contraceptive methods are pursued and that condoms are used for safer sex (Local Authorities Associations' Officer Working Group on AIDS, 1989). In developing countries, 'women may be burdened with the responsibility of changing things over which they have little influence and less control' (Mahmoud, deZalduondo and Zewdie, 1990).

To date most of the evidence suggests that HIV is more likely to be transmitted from male clients to prostitutes than the other way around (Cohen, Alexander and Wofsy, 1988; Khabbaz *et al.*, 1990). Whether or not women who are injecting drug users are also prostitutes is not the real issue in the debates about the transmission of HIV. For women the real issue is how the HIV/AIDS issue is being used to scapegoat, criminalise or victimise individual women, believed to be from high-risk groups of polluted women.

While AIDS is a matter of life and death, there is a need for more women to speak out and to expose how they are targeted as a social group (see, for example, Rieder and Ruppelt, 1989). In effect women who inject drugs and female prostitutes tend to be lumped together into high-risk groups. This is particularly revealing when one considers evidence suggesting that a very high percentage of heterosexual women with AIDS (72 per cent) were infected by injecting drug users, most probably heterosexual or bisexual men (US Department of Health and Human Services, 1986). The following statement from organised, western prostitutes clarifies this issue:

> The small minority of prostitutes who are needle-using drug addicts are at risk from shared needles, not from commercial sex . . . Prostitution is not responsible for drug addiction. (International Committee for Prostitutes' Rights, 1987)

One could also say that drug addiction is not responsible for prostitution, a fact that tends to remain hidden in the literature on both HIV/AIDS and drug use. Furthermore a study on drug-addicted prostitutes reports that 'prostitution does not constitute an additional risk factor' when women are injecting drug users (Dan, Rock and Bar-Shani, 1987).

Prostitutes may be more at risk from having sex with injecting drug users who may also be their regular sexual partners than from being 'on the game'. But, as Padian (1988) points out, we do not know the relative risk of needle sharing versus sexual contacts with infected partners. Also, no one has yet expressed concern that prostitutes might get AIDS from their male customers (Alexander, 1987).

Arguing within a feminist perspective, Lynne Segal (1989) highlights the anti-sex rhetoric linked with the public reaction to AIDS and notes that AIDS has not been taken up as a feminist issue. She argues that the WLM (Women's Liberation Movement) has effected a long battle 'for women's control of their own sexuality'. The goal for women was 'to be free to choose when and if to have a child . . . and to obtain sexual pleasure free from fears of pregnancy, disease and male coercion'. Segal implies that AIDS and feminism do not mix. This is because, at a point when women were exploring sexual pleasure and demanding it for its own sake, AIDS came onto the scene. In the face of the virus, women's sexual explorations came to a halt.

On the other hand, it could be argued that the exploration of sexual pleasure, highlighted by Segal, is limited. This is because privileged women, white, heterosexual, middle-class and professionals, are seen to be the main agents engaged in this sexual exploration. Black women, poor women, drug-using women, prostitutes, lesbians or any group of women with a minority voice and less social power tend to be excluded from this form of 'sex intellectualising'. AIDS has consistently been a feminist issue. That the voices of women with less access to social power have not been heard is perhaps more a result of deep divisions amongst women than of AIDS being an uncomfortable topic for white, middle-class women. If the AIDS message is anti-sex, this is because women want to continue exploring sexual pleasure without confronting their own anxieties with regard to safer, heterosexual sex. Either they would like pleasure without traditional penetrative sex, or at some level, sex without a condom, the primary accoutrement of safer penetrative sex. For other, less privileged women (such as a prostitute in sub-Saharan Africa) a condom may be viewed as a luxury product, while exploring sexual pleasure may not exist as an option in their lives.

AIDS is very much a feminist issue. As Alexander (1987) argues, feminists need to know the facts and 'to exert leadership in dealing with the disease without blaming its victims'. Simply, feminists should be concerned for every woman's welfare: for drug users, prostitutes and other stigmatised groups of woman with HIV infection in both developed and developing countries.

In this context, it is important to know that, in the interests of public health, female prostitutes are being increasingly observed by 'caring' researchers, fieldworkers and health workers. There is very little if any discussion about the intrusion into the private lives of these women. Indeed the fact that prostitutes have private lives tends to be overlooked (Day and Ward, 1990) in most research. Related to this research issue, addiction experts/researchers have moved swiftly into the HIV/AIDS area to colonise new groups of captive populations in the 'sex industry' for their 'scientific work'. (For examples, see Thomas, Plant, Plant and Sales, 1989; Plant 1990.)

Additionally work with women prostitutes and women drug users is becoming increasingly fashionable, regardless of the fact that one may encounter real human suffering, pain and deprivation in this type of research. One has a sense at times that 'social scientific' work with drug-using prostitutes is viewed, in the eyes of some researchers, as glamorous. Perhaps academic careers and the need for future funding from government sources are viewed as more important than the public/sex work and private/sex lives of these 'minority' women. If this is the case, research observations and professional interests appear to take priority over the lives of what researchers observe: real human subjects – prostitute women.

As a result of this type of research, more control and surveillance has been exerted over the lives of women who are, in society's eyes, social outcasts and workers within an emerging underclass of oppressed people. In recent years, women prostitutes have generated an awareness of safer sex/work practices on a public scale (English Collective of Prostitutes, 1987). They have created for themselves more space than ever before for organising women sex workers on an international level (Delacoste and Alexander, 1987).

It is ironic that in resisting the virus these women have not resisted and in some instances allowed members of the scientific community access to information about intimate details of both their public and private lives. At the time as prostitutes finally achieved a certain amount of professional power, what Day (1988) identifies as professionalisation, male-defined professionals under the guise of AIDS prevention have gained access to prostitutes' work space. These professional workers, with or without a voyeuristic gaze, attempt to help prostitutes protect themselves from the risks of catching the virus. From another standpoint it could be argued that they are protecting themselves and hetero-sexual men. As Alexander (1987, p. 260) suggests, 'when women or gay/bisexual men get AIDS, it's their fault, but if heterosexual men come down with the disease, it is the fault of women and gay/ bisexual men'. In this context the women are prostitutes and drug users.

In conclusion, this chapter has looked critically at some of the false images and beliefs which surround women's use of an illegal drug, heroin. While heroin may be seen as a masculine drug, women who use heroin, like their non-heroin using counterparts, are expected to be dependent on men, male partners or male society. As polluted women, heroin users are seen to spoil their identities as well as their private and public lives. If they seek treatment they are treated less well than men. Furthermore the drug treatment system, in order to offer a comprehensive response to women must consider the needs of special groups of women, such as black women, lesbians. Significantly we have seen that AIDS has had an impact upon women, particularly injecting drug users and prostitutes.

It is hoped that the discussions in this chapter have demonstrated why women and heroin use is a feminist issue. More insights need to be developed in order to give hope to women who at the present time are unable to stop using heroin. Women-oriented treatment and research environments that are both intellectually sensitive and caring towards women need to be nurtured. Finally within these environments the consciousness of women drug users needs to be raised, as these women emerge from their despair and isolation.

5

Women and smoking

When Belphoebe finds Timices sorely wounded she enters into the wood
to seek for herbs:
There whether it divine Tabacco were,
Or Panachea or Polygony,
She found and brought it to her patient deare. (*Fairie Queen*)

The patient dear is Sir Walter Raleigh (A. Chute, 1961 *Tabacco*, edited
by F. P. Wilson (Oxford: Basil Blackwell).

Introduction

There is conflicting evidence about the term 'tobacco' and its
origins. Whether it originated from the name of the island,
Tobago, one of the Caribbean islands north of the equator, where
evidence of tobacco cultivation has existed since 1493 or from the
Spanish name of the province of Tobaco in the Yukatan Peninsula
in Southeast Mexico is unclear (Brooks, 1953, p. 65). Nevertheless
the most cultivated species of tobacco, Nicotiana rustica and
Nicotiana tabacum, have been smoked, drunk, licked, snuffed and
chewed for thousands of years (Koskowski, 1955). Their use in pre-
European times has been traced to various cultures including the
Incas of Peru, West Indians and Central, North and South
American Indians.

While drinking tobacco appears to be the most ancient method of
administration, drawing in and puffing out smoke is the most
common method in society today. In this light, Russell (1974) has
identified tobacco smoking as 'the most addictive and dependence-
producing form of object specific self-administered gratification

known to man [sic]' and recently the implications of tobacco use as drug addiction has been outlined quite comprehensively (United States Department of Health and Human Services, 1988).

On a global scale cigarette smoking accounts for tens of millions of deaths and its growth has been identified in epidemic proportions (WHO, 1979). In the developed world, smoking-related disease has increased at a phenomenal rate, particularly amongst women, while tremendous concentration of economic power in the few, large multinational companies presents a formidable obstacle to any attempts by governments or individuals to control this development.

Bobbie Jacobson, in her books, *The Ladykillers: Why Smoking is a Feminist Issue* (1981) and *Beating the Ladykillers: Women and Smoking* (1986), develops a very valuable framework in this area. For her, smoking is emblematic of women's subordinate status and inferiority. In this context she says (1986, p. 111):

Smoking is an outward sign of our [women's] constant battle to control our unvoiced frustrations; controlling these means we can be 'nice' to everybody all the time. To feel in control of our lives is just as important to men as it is to us, but the ways to exert this control open to us are more limited. We will tolerate unruly or drunken husbands or angry bosses who take it out on us, but who can we take it out on? Surely not our children. So we reach for the cigarette instead.

This chapter attempts to extend the feminist framework in this area, while uncovering some of the invisible social issues that are related to women's use of cigarettes. The main operating assumption of this chapter is twofold: women use cigarettes differently from men and the reasons for these differences are based on women's social positioning or 'the politics of women's social position' (Randall, 1987). Developing a critical analysis of women's smoking, sensitive to the structural issues of class, race and gender will be undertaken.

A review of the clinical literature on smoking reveals that over the past 20 years there has been a plethora of work in the substance use field on smoking and disease, the physiological and psychological factors related to smoking, the effects of a variety of treatment regimes and smoking cessation rates. While smoking and pregnancy has emerged increasingly as an area of concern, it is important to ensure that concern is motivated by humane, compassionate responses rather informed by moralistic attitudes (DAWN, 1988b).

In recent years clinicians and researchers in the field have focused more attention on women than they did in the past. However work on women smokers tends to be framed within a male-centred approach. To paint a clear picture of women's smoking is to clarify the sorts of issues which need to be included within a framework which is sensitive to women. Keeping one's feminist eyes open, one needs to make links between women's smoking and 'gender-illuminating notions' such as dependency, labour, caring and pleasure. In the following discussions illustrative material is presented with these links in mind. As a result key structural concerns related to the progression of smoking as a feminist issue will be highlighted.

A view of the tobacco industry

On a global scale the tobacco industry, one of the world's most profitable industries, is made up of some of the most powerful multinational companies including Philip Morris Incorporated (USA), R. J. Reynolds Inc. (USA), American Brands Inc. (USA), British–American Tobacco Industries (UK), the Imperial Group (UK) and the Rembrandt Group (South Africa). Taylor (1984, p. xviii) points out that, as commodities, cigarettes are inexpensive to produce, highly addictive and 'recession proof'.

In Britain, ASH (Action on Smoking and Health, 1990a) noted that in 1988–9 the Treasury earned £6040 million in revenue from tobacco duty and that tobacco is the third largest source of consumer revenue. The tobacco industry has annual sales of four trillion cigarettes worth over $40 billion (Taylor, 1984, p. xviii) making the industry 'dependent' on cigarettes, as is the smoker.

The industry spends a considerable amount on sales promotion through advertising and gift coupons. In the last 20 years new forms of promotion have included sponsorship of sports events such as the Embassy World Professional Snooker Championship, Virginia Slims Tennis Circuit and the Benson and Hedges Tennis Championship as well as artistic endeavours (the John Player portrait awards and the Benson and Hedges Music Festival at Adleburgh). While sponsorship of sports and the arts grew about 20 per cent a year in the 1970s, the £15 million spent in 1973 had risen to £50 million by 1981 (Wilkinson, 1986).

The 'women's market' has been specifically exploited by the industry with the development of cigarettes designed specifically for women (Eve, Virginia Slims, Kim and Silva Thins) along with increased spending on advertising in women's magazines. Between 1977 and 1984 spending in women's magazines rose 50 per cent to £4.5 million and by 1984 the tobacco industry had spent nearly £7 million annually. Besides aiming at women, the industry has seen developing countries as relatively new gainful markets.

In the 1960s tobacco production in developing countries contributed 17 per cent to the total world production of tobacco; by 1976 this had increased to 40 per cent. Today tobacco is grown in more than 120 countries, the majority of which are developing countries. While world production of tobacco increased by 42 per cent between 1961 and 1984, the share of world tobacco leaf output grown in less developed countries increased from about 50 per cent to over 60 per cent between 1965 and 1984 (Powell, 1989). Jacobson (1985) found that developing countries consumed more than half of all the world's tobacco and that the 2.1 per cent annual rise in global cigarette consumption was mostly within third-world countries.

A report by Ruth Roemer (1982) under the auspices of the World Health Organisation has criticised the tobacco industry for destroying efforts to decrease the world's smoking consumption. She says:

> The tremendous concentration of economic power in the seven transnational tobacco conglomerates presents a formidable obstacle to governments struggling to discourage their young people from taking up smoking and to persuade smokers to free themselves from tobacco dependence. Ranged on the side of the tobacco interests are their enormous financial resources, their control of industrial technology for producing, manufacturing and packaging tobacco products, their mastery of sophisticated marketing techniques and their secret weapon – the addictive nature of tobacco.

While governments do not have secret weapons to combat the smoking problem, the annual revenue that the state receives from cigarettes can be seen as an embarrassing paradox. For governments the clear economic advantages of cigarette consumption may be seen to take priority over the somewhat hidden disadvantages or what have been referred to as the private and social costs of smoking (Markandya and Pearce, 1989). Revenue from cigarettes is a source of funds to help reduce deficits and in Britain a 20 per cent reduction in smoking would lead to an increased trade deficit of £50 million at the end of a five-year period (Taylor, 1984, p. 72).

In the United States in the mid-1970s the economic consequences of smoking were estimated to be $27 500 million, including $8200 million for direct health care costs (Roemer, 1982). As stated previously, in Britain revenue from cigarettes brings the Chancellor of the Exchequer £6 billion per annum while it has been estimated that cigarette-related diseases cost the NHS £500 million a year (ASH, 1990a). On the one hand, the activities of the tobacco industry (producing and distributing cigarettes) promote a serious health dilemma; on the other, these activities have an important economic function in society.

Tobacco consumption and women as active consumers

In 1950, Doll and Hill (1950) published the results of an epidemiological study which made clear links between smoking and lung cancer. Since that time there have been many attempts by policy makers, the medical profession, researchers and health educators to generate a public awareness of the damage that smoking does to one's health. In 1962, 1971, 1977 and 1983, the Royal College of Physicians published a series of reports on smoking, representing clear statements on the public health dangers of smoking. Their 1983 report, *Health or Smoking?*, noted that since the 1970s the issue of women and smoking was one of the most important developments in smoking research.

Few women in Britain smoked before the First World War (Royal College of Physicians, 1977); in the USA the development of the blended cigarette in 1913 was preparing the way for the extensive use of smoking by women (Wagner, 1971). Before the Second World War smoking was considered unfeminine and comments such as 'Smoking is something nice girls don't do' were the order of the day (Montross and Montross, 1923, p. 245).

In 1930 it was estimated that 2 per cent of the US adult population of smokers were women over 18 years of age, while this figure rose steadily to 39 per cent by 1961 (Burbank, 1972).

Jacobson (1981, p. 11) noted that in 1950 the average British woman got through half as many cigarettes as men smokers, but by the late 1970s she caught up and smoked more than 15 cigarettes a day. Jacobson also pointed out that women in the late 1970s smoked more heavily than their equals in the 1950s and, perhaps more importantly, that they were younger. In 1982, a cross-national study of young people suggested that more girls than boys may be smoking between the ages of 13 and 16 (Aaro, Wood, Kanner and Rimpela, 1984). For boys and girls aged 11 to 16, more recent figures suggest that, by 1986, 7 per cent of boys and 12 per cent of girls smoked. In 1988, boys smoking remained at 7 per cent but girls still smoked more, at 9 per cent (ASH, 1990b).

The Institute for the Study of Drug Dependence (ISDD, 1987) points out that since the early 1950s, when 60 per cent of men and 40 per cent of women smoked, the percentage of smokers has decreased but, until recently, the individual smoker was smoking more, with the result that the total number of cigarettes smoked each year was growing. The Royal College of Physicians (1983, p. 62) reported that women aged between 20 and 59 were 'the heaviest female smokers' in Britain. Jacobson (1986, p. 7) identifies US female smokers as 'the world's heaviest smokers' with the proportion of women in the United States smoking heavily having more than doubled since 1965.

Given the above, it is interesting to look at overall prevalence in the United States and Britain and to see that the gap which once existed between men and women smokers has narrowed. Observing the British situation, ISDD (1987, p. 10) points out that 'from 20 to 60 years of age the prevalence of smoking is more or less constant at around 40% for men and 36% for women decreasing to 30% for men and 23% for women aged 60 or more'. Schuman (1978) found that, in the United States, there had been a gradual decline between 1964 and 1975 in the percentage of men who were smokers (52 per cent to 39 per cent) but there had been little change for women (31 per cent to 28 per cent). Official US statistics (USDHHS, 1989) show that, in 1983, 35 per cent of men aged over 20 and 27 per cent of women of the same age group smoked. By 1987, these figures were 32 per cent and 27 per cent respectively.

With 14 million smokers in Britain (half of them women), the picture for women is bleak: both the proportion of women smoking and the amount they smoke has been nearing those for men

(Jacobson, 1986, p. 5). In 1986, 35 per cent of men and 31 per cent of women smoked. In 1988, the figures were 33 per cent and 30 per cent (ASH, 1990c). On a global scale, the decline in smoking is greater for men than for women, suggesting that smoking is a bigger problem for women. For example, in Finland, where smoking has been identified as 'the single most important preventable cause of death', the proportion of men smoking since the 1960s has remained steady at about 35 per cent, while for women the proportion has gradually increased from about 16 per cent to 20 per cent (Pekurinen, 1989).

The symbols of smoking in the public and the private spheres

It would be useful at this point to focus attention on issues which tend to remain invisible in the women and smoking debate and to look at the subtleties involved.

The politics of gender can be seen to be operating soon after tobacco became a commodity. For example, in Britain, James I waged the first known 'war against tobacco' when he published *Counterblaste to Tobacco*, in 1604. Jeger (1965) points out that James I and his supporters, outraged by the unproductive tendencies of young 'English gallants', believed them to be risking their masculinity by smoking. Jeger (1965, p. 76) cites the appropriate text in *Counterblaste to Tobacco*:

> Tobacco the outlandish weed,
> It spends the brain and spoils the seed.
> It dulls the sprite, it dims the sight,
> It robs a woman of her right.

The message is that men become impotent ('spoils the seed'), thus stealing from women ('robs a woman') their 'right' to strong, manly males. In effect men, using tobacco, were viewed as effete, weak, unspritely and 'feminised' men.

Interestingly enough a similar theme emerged more than 200 years later, when cigarettes were introduced before the American Civil War. At first they were seen as 'effeminate' because of their less powerful quality (that is, immediate effect) than pipe smoking, snuffing tobacco or chewing tobacco (Robert, 1952). For a man, to smoke cigarettes was to be seen to be feminine, but this image had to be changed, given that 'a number of Federal tobacco taxes, including a tax on cigarettes were imposed in 1864 as part of a package of taxes to finance the Civil War' (Lewitt, 1989, p. 1217). Cigarette smoking became linked to the perpetuation of a war economy and more acceptable as a male activity. While men were able to smoke publicly, women tended to smoke in private (Robert, 1952). What had previously been viewed as effeminate activity gradually became 'masculinised' by the war. As MacDonald (1987, p. 9) suggests, 'when war intrudes into society . . . it may be very difficult to maintain the traditional social order and boundaries such as those of gender may well break down'.

There is no clear evidence on whether or not smoking became predominantly a male activity in the late nineteenth and early twentieth centuries. As early as 1885, tobacco was identified as an enemy of women, suggesting perhaps increased male smoking activity. Gritz (1980, p. 492), quoting from M. Lander's work, *The Tobacco Problem*, published in 1885, notes that tobacco was seen as the persistent foe of woman, 'isolating woman from her society . . . marring, if not positively undermining the relations between the sexes'.

As one of the first commodities to be taxed in North America (Lewitt, 1989), tobacco became an essential requirement for the generation of substantial revenue for the United States Federal government. The social relations of the production and consumption of tobacco took priority over what was seen as the 'damaging' effect on the social relations between the sexes. Perhaps this was easy to justify, given that this 'damaging effect' was occasioned in the private sphere, a sphere over which men were already beginning to exert control.

Smoking and poverty

Regardless of whether or not cigarettes are viewed as socially damaging, they are a commodity as well as a legal drug. This drug is produced, distributed and sold for vast profits. It is consumed for a variety of social, psychological and emotional reasons by millions of men and women of all social classes in developed and developing countries, yet of the seven million women who smoke in Britain, 60 per cent are women in working-class households (Graham, 1987).

Graham (1983, p. 23) asserts that the rise of capitalism and its attendant sexual division of labour is linked to the social and spatial separation of production from reproduction. With this separation, the social organisation of caring falls primarily within the reproductive, private sphere and squarely upon women's shoulders in the family. Ultimately 'caring' describes the specific kind of 'privatised' labour women perform in society.

Within this framework Graham mounted a study of women caring for pre-school children in order to explore the day-to-day realities of informal health care. From this larger study she looked at a group of mothers from low-income families caring for pre-school children and she had a particular concern for the impact of poverty and single parenthood on the caring responsibilities of these women.

She found that smoking for women functions both as a necessity and a luxury when material and human resources are limited (Graham, 1987). As a necessity, it helps women to structure caring and/or to reintroduce structure into their labour routine when it starts breaking down. Smoking becomes a way of coping with stress, motherhood and women's experience of poverty. In a real sense, it is a specific work strategy, linked to the efficient production of domestic labour for these women. As a luxury, smoking is a leisure activity, the relatively small space between her experience of alienated and non-alienated caring; it represents a space and time for mother to look after herself rather than her children. In this way it becomes a woman's real taking of space for herself.

In this theoretical framework the woman smoker, whether she smokes to structure her caring (as a necessity) or to relax (as a luxury), is displaying a form of self-management, control and decision making in the private sphere. Objectively she can be seen as an active consumer. She is not only attempting to impose order on a somewhat chaotic way of life in the private world of children, house and family, but also asserting herself, actively taking space from her mundane social existence and performing a major self-directed activity.

Similar to the woman tranquilliser user, she may be in a structurally powerless position, but for the woman smoker this lack of power is related to her status of poverty rather than to her status as wife and patient *vis-à-vis* her husband and her doctor. Unlike the women tranquilliser user, the woman smoker is not 'strung-out patient' or 'dutiful wife' managed and manageable in an environment legitimated by male authority. The woman smoker, in this light, perceives herself as coping, in control and a good mother. Her 'nicotine fix' is related to her autonomy as well as her dependence on living in poverty. Smoking expresses her independence in the midst of dependency. Her dependency 'of the addiction kind' appears to take priority over her dependency 'of the subordinate thing kind'. Given that smoking can be described as one of the diseases of affluence, emerging from the rich world (Seager and Olson, 1986), it is rather ironic that it is a practice linked not only with women from low-income families but also with their way of coping with poverty.

Smoking is also related to the way that, with the social and spatial separation of production from reproduction, a woman smoker is attempting to make a distinction between work and leisure in the private sphere, 'a distinction that is generally much less clear for women than for men' (Leonard and Speakman, 1986, p. 26). In this context her drug is indeed a recreational drug, a 'smoke ring of pleasure'.

On the other hand, while cigarettes as a necessity can be 'her symbol of participation in an adult, consumer society' (Graham, 1987), that society is ultimately public, male-directed and male-oriented, a potential threat to the creation and extension of her much-needed private, female, space. While cigarettes have become an economic necessity in global terms, a woman's participation in consuming this necessity not only damages her health but also has the potential, if she develops any smoking-related diseases, to put her into a category of ill health where she is blamed for her illness.

Lesley Doyal (1981, p. 34) suggests that what is referred to in the health literature as 'way of life factors' – including diet, stress, smoking and lack of exercise – are crucial in causing a 'new disease burden'. She argues that 'ill health' is now being explained in terms of 'individual moral failings – by blaming the victims for what has happened to them'. Similarly Thunhurst (1982, p. 25) contends that the overconsumption of tobacco should be seen properly as 'a common symptom of stress rather than wayward habits that people in their foolishness choose to adopt'. Yet the hidden factor remains: while cigarettes are an essential part of the ebb and flow of government's fiscal requirements, the woman smoker becomes the victim of this invisible need for increased revenue.

Smoking and ethnicity

The smoking picture appears to differ for black women and white women. Rates of smoking are much lower for Asian and Afro-Caribbean women than among white women in Britain (Graham, 1987); in the United States the gap between white women and black woman is smaller (USDHHS, 1989). One British study (Gabe and Thorogood, 1986b) suggests that, in comparison to white working-class women, black working-class women with poorer housing, greater domestic burdens and little leisure activities did not smoke as much. Having limited leisure activity as a result of exhaustion, the black women reported a series of alternative resources (other than substance use) which helped them to cope: religion, paid work and close relationships with their children, particularly daughters.

Bryan, Dadzie and Scafe (1985, p. 124), discussing the experiences of Afro-Caribbean women, emphasise that black women have consistently been active in their communities and that this activity has been focused on 'the formation of small church, social and welfare groups which represent a spontaneous response to the isolation and alienation Black women face' in a white racist society. In a related context, they point out that the dynamics of the Afro-Caribbean family structure based on kinship relations and communalism has enabled a 'common respect for women' and a recognition of 'the important role mothers play in the social, political and economic life of the community' (p. 183). Mirroring these ideas, Carby (1982, p. 231) notes that there are 'strong female support networks which exist in both West Indian and Asian sex/gender systems' and that the existence of these female networks means that black women are key figures in the development of survival strategies.

Black women in Britain, with strong kinship bonds as well as private and public support networks, create effective 'social and psychological buffers', acting as survival strategies in the face of isolation, poverty and the experience of racism. Black women appear to have the experience of greater autonomy in the private sphere than white women which enables them to use the other resources besides smoking to cope with their everyday lives, which were identified in Gabe and Thorogood's (1986) study. There appears to be less of a need for black women to structure their caring through smoking. When they need to release themselves from the stresses of the home, they may shift their energies into paid work in the public sphere, although they tend to fare less well than white women (Brown, 1984). On the other hand, they may find work in the private sphere of domestic service where social relations mirror very clearly divisions of gender, class and race (Graham, 1991). Their public paid work, primarily in the services sector, is 'little more than institutionalised housework' (Bryan, Dadzie and Scafe, 1985, p. 25), reflecting their experience of unpaid labour in the private sphere.

Regardless of their involvement in paid work, black women, like all women, experience the need for a distinction between work and leisure in the private sphere. However, this distinction appears to be less clear within their gendered households. Whether or not this implies that leisure as a resource is less available to them, as Gabe and Thorogood suggest (1986b, p. 755), black women's poverty tends to propel them into paid work rather than smoking or other forms of substance use. In this way paid work may be more of a survival strategy than a resource. More significantly, through this survival strategy, black women may be experiencing harm equal to or more damaging than the harm experienced by their smoking counterparts.

> For the majority of Black women . . . It has been night and shift work which have enabled us to carry out our responsibilities as mothers and breadwinners. Inadequate sleep, exhaustion and ill-health were the price we have had to pay if we wanted to spend time with our children and feed them too – even when we weren't struggling to do it alone. (Bryan, Dadzie and Scafe, 1985, p. 31)

It is difficult to get a picture of smoking *vis-à-vis* black women in the United States. This is primarily because large-scale studies (Johnson, O'Malley, Bachman, 1987; Ravcis and Kandel, 1987) tend to ignore the issue of race, racism and their effects on social behaviour. If race is a key variable, as in a massive study of 111 024 patients in the San Francisco Bay area (Seltzer, Friedman and Siegelaub, 1974), it is difficult to consider seriously findings which speak of 'black, white and yellow female smokers'. Black women and white women have had similar prevalence rates in the USA (USDHEW, 1980) and recent 1987 statistics put both groups at 27.9 per cent and 27.3 per cent respectively (USDHHS, 1989). However overall female smoking has been found to be related to family income, with women in higher-income families (excluding professional women) smoking more (Gritz, 1980). This is not a true picture of all women, given that a distinction between one-income and two-income families is not made in these statistics. That there exists a wide gap in research on differences between black women and white women's smoking evidences the need for more work in this area. There is a need to shift emphasis in the public health field to consider the subtle effects of racism *vis-à-vis* substance use in both the public and private lives of black women.

Research in the United States is currently centred on 'topical' substances such as cocaine (including crack) and opiates rather than on less emotionally inflammatory substances such as nicotine. Given the increasing focus on illegal drug use as a cause of increased urban disintegration and malaise, this is not surprising. While the war on drugs has not included tobacco, young black men are increasingly the target as this war is waged. For black Americans, smoking may be perceived as a somewhat minor health or welfare issue in the face of the overwhelming social problems of police harassment, poverty, homelessness or involvement with illegal drugs. In this context it is ironic that dependence on slavery ('free black labour') was essential for the development of commercial agriculture in the Southern United States and Virginian tobacco plantations played a major role in this economic development in the run-up to the US Civil war (Moore, 1966).

A feminist view: smoking, pleasure and pain

The last section of this chapter attempts to develop a women-oriented view of smoking as a form of substance use for women. Smoking can be seen as a habit while habit is defined as a settled tendency or practice. Smoking for women can be seen in this light as a female settled tendency or practice. It is a habit linked to dependency both of 'a subordinate thing kind' and of 'an addiction kind'. In order to make valuable links with feminist theory, this discussion begins with a women-centred conception, emphasising women's praxis. This conception reflects a feminist principle, put forward in an eloquent paper, 'Women's Work: Women's Knowledge' by Hilary Rose (1986b). In this work, Hilary Rose maintains that there is an integral need for women to see their existence, their very materiality in the 'masculinist' world as rooted in their own everyday lived experiences. While upholding a feminist epistemology, she demonstrates how women's caring is deeply connected to women's labour. In turn, she challenges the view that women's caring labour is merely a 'piece' of the formation of the female identity. She says:

> A feminist epistemology derives from women's lived experiences, centred on the domains of interconnectedness and affectual rationality. It emphasizes holism and harmonious relationships with nature . . . Feminist knowledge transcends masculinist knowledge . . . (pp. 162–3)

In a related context, she says:

> As a profoundly sensuous activity, women's labour constitutes a material reality which structures a distinctive understanding of the social and natural worlds (p. 171)

As we have seen from earlier discussions in this chapter, smoking for women represents a somewhat active strategy connected with women's labour and leisure. Whether or not it is viewed as unhealthy, it is perceived as a permissible activity which tends to affirm the very materiality of a woman's body and to validate the substance of her labour. As a sensuous subject, a woman smoker may fluctuate between an identity of 'a woman who is capable of experiencing pleasure' and an identity of an angry, frustrated, devalued and bored carer. In a very real sense, her private pleasure is born out of a shared, social or 'patriarchal' pain with other carers like herself. This patriarchal pain refers to any of a number of distressing ordeals women experience both publicly and privately in a gendered system of domination. Patriarchal pain is the direct result of the myriad politics of women's social positioning. (This notion will be discussed further in Chapter 7.)

Recently, in the field of substance use, Dorn and South (1989), discussing young people's illegal drug use (heroin) and the effects of this upon family life, contend that the social problem of drug use illustrates the complex intermixing of pleasure and constraint: in the context of the family, drug use necessitates the recognition that individual pleasure is closely linked with social pain.

Although smoking is not an illegal activity, links with the above-mentioned work can be useful in developing a feminist analysis. An interesting standpoint on smoking and women can be created within the 'feminist prism of women's praxis', refracting Dorn and South's 'gender-sensitive' formula. For example, that smoking for some women helps to create a sense of pleasure, delight and satisfaction in gendered workaday lives, more often than not filled with caring for others, children, housework and stress, is worthy of exploration.

Smoking for pleasure may be conscious or an awareness of pleasure may remain below the surface of any woman's interconnectedness with her sensuous self, yet many women smoke because they enjoy it as a pleasurable sensation and all women need pleasure. In this context work carried out by experts in the field of smoking (Ashton and Stepney, 1982) suggests 'that the most important single factor in the whole smoking phenomenon is that smoking is pleasurable to smokers; they like doing it' (p. 54). While smoking may not be pleasurable at all times, 'it gives enough pleasure to override the concomitant unpleasant sensations' (p. 54). In an interesting discussion on the pharmacology of smoking, these authors point out how nicotine as a drug acts not only on 'pleasure centres' but also 'punishment pathways' in the brain. In other words, while nicotine stimulates pleasure sensations, it can also inhibit nerve cell responses (synapses) in these 'punishment pathways'. As regards the latter response, doses of nicotine administered through smoking cigarettes have marked effects in 'allaying unpleasant emotions, such as anxiety, fear, boredom, frustration and anger' (p. 56). In a slightly different light, smoking inhibits 'punishment pathways' as well as being experienced as pleasurable.

Another author (Bejerot, 1980) refers to dependence on nicotine as 'nicotinism' and suggests that all drug addiction is a 'chemical love'. Describing this chemical love, he says:

> The pleasure mechanism may be stimulated in a number of ways and give rise to a strong fixation on repetitive behaviour . . . The simplest way of regarding drug addiction is to see it as falling in love with specific, pleasurable sensations (or the means to prevent pain). (p. 254)

While findings in this area of work on neurotransmitters *vis-à-vis* nicotine remain inconclusive, a fuller understanding of the women and smoking issue can be had by considering how smoking performs a similar 'social' function for women: we see that smoking as substance use highlights the fact that women need to allow themselves to seek pleasure and to avoid unpleasant, strong, perhaps uncontrollable emotions. While smoking is a form of enjoyment or even a 'chemical love' in a woman's life somewhat devoid of leisure and/or leisure time, it is also an effective way of appeasing unpleasant feelings.

Smoking serves to block out all sorts of self-punishing feelings a woman may be feeling as an individual trapped in a well defined social space. On the one hand, within this space she confronts herself and her caring labour extracted for dependent others; on the other, she experiences a need to extract herself, her independent self, for 'a smoke ring of pleasure'. In this light, smoking is a diversion if not an escape from patriarchal pain, the series of contradictory, unpleasant emotions experienced in and through the inescapable struggle between masculinist reality and women's praxis. It could be suggested further that all substance use for women has elements of this theme, if only in seed form.

As the issue of smoking is linked with women's praxis, the need for broad conceptions of substance use, inclusive of structural issues such as race, class and gender, becomes apparent. Linking an understanding of women's praxis to the smoking issue uncovers powerful ideologies and practices which are directed at women smokers. While it appears that smoking serves different as well as similar social and psychological functions for men and women, it is nevertheless a feminist issue. Along with Jacobson (1986, p. 108), this author shares the view that smoking as a feminist issue *is not* a matter of claiming that 'the rise of smoking amongst women over the last 15 years is a consequence of the parallel rise of the feminist movement of the 1960s'.

The quest for women's liberation is not one of striving for power and competitiveness *vis-à-vis* men. Women's liberation is concerned with the way women's praxis offers a transformative way of thinking, feeling and acting in women's public and private space. That notions of pleasure, dependency, caring, labour, social space, power and women's praxis have all been identified as gender-illuminating notions with regard to women's smoking suggests that there needs to be a transformative shift within work carried out by women and for women in the substance use field. Women smokers need to feel that, while smoking may be experienced as a 'piece' of their immediate 'inferiority reduction', this effect does not last. Women smokers finding themselves caught between their caring labour as burden and as a source of self-fulfilment may need a vision. This vision includes a new conception of their labour rooted in what Meis (1986, p. 217) calls the 'production of immediate life in all its aspects':

> A feminist conception of labour has to be oriented towards the production of life as the goal of work and not the production of things and wealth . . . It has, therefore, to be oriented towards a different concept of time, in which time is not segregated into portions of burdensome labour and portions of supposed pleasure and leisure, but in which times of work and times of rest and enjoyment are alternating and interspersed . . . even a lifetime of work will not then be felt as a curse but as a source of human fulfilment and happiness . . . [this] cannot be brought about unless the existing sexual division of labour is abolished. (p. 217)

To nurture this vision women need to create a vision of themselves not only as carers but also as enablers, allowing a sense of well-being for themselves and for others. While smoking is disabling, it appears to give some women a grounding in pleasure. Being mindful of the differences of race, class, culture, age, sexual orientation and ableness amongst them, women need to look at the way in which 'the production of immediate life in all aspects' can replace a pleasurable routine, smoking, with life-giving rather than life-threatening practices.

A way forward requires that women smokers recognise that in some sense they have 'captured lungs' as well as 'captured wombs' (Oakley, 1984). Perhaps women smokers need to find more space for women's praxis, and to breathe 'women-centred' sighs of relief may be part of this recognition. Women require strategies or alternative resources to fill this gap in their need for pleasure without damaging their health. But for some women this task is perhaps insurmountable, given the contradictions they face between caring for others and caring for themselves. It has already been shown that smoking serves to provide positive nurturing or 'strokes' on an emotional level in both aspects of caring. This demonstrates that women need to live in a society where these emotional strokes are easily available to them as women, where their dependence upon caring does not foster dependence upon drugs and where pleasure is a matter of access to life not death or inhaling nicotine, as well as other dangerous substances such as carbon monoxide, ammonia, DDT, tars, cadmium and radioactivity (Stepney, 1987, p. 14).

More importantly women need to live in a society where women's labour as a direct sensual interaction with the material world is freely given, valued and reciprocated. There is a need for a world free from patriarchal pain and centred on female as well as male authenticity. Women have a right to name their experiences and not to see them lost in a 'cloud of smoke'.

We may conclude with a brief reference to creative imagery, which will allow some readers to explore at a deeper, women-oriented level the more invisible issues related to women and smoking. Some feminists find pleasure in creative imagery as they search for their 'elemental praxis' or women-centred roots. In this search they attempt to validate themselves, their material reality, their labour and their love.

For women, fire and smoke have traditionally been symbols of mystical power. In the realm of myth, Daly (1988) identifies women's praxis as mediated by fire and developed by a wisdom which 'burns away the mindbindings of psychic numbing' (p. 159). In this context, Daly suggests that women need deep wisdom enabling them 'to rise like Phoenixes from the ashes of the Atrocious State' (p. 158). The implication here is that women in touch with their Female Selves need to create a world that enables them to rise from a gendered system of domination, not a world in which cigarette ash and all that it represents falls from women's fingertips.

Additionally, within the context of current feminist mythology, the image of the Salamander is one of a female fire spirit who has the power to endure fire and smoke without harm. She is a 'Dragon-identified' woman. However, regardless of whether or not women want to be 'dragon-identified' at a psychic level, do women, like 'real' dragons, need to have smoke coming out of their nostrils? We must hope that, for increasing numbers of women, the answer to this question will be 'no'.

6

Women and food dependence

. . . the space of a silhouette
entering the space of silence . . .
the woman who walks beyond
the streets of desire
the womon who has always walked these streets
with passion
the womon who has taken over the space of her body
and the womon who has refused to conquer that space . . .
('whoever i am i'm a fat woman', Sharon Bas Hannah)

Introduction

This chapter focuses on women's somewhat problematic relationship to food and develops a feminist analysis of women's use and
misuse of food or addiction to food. As we know from previous
chapters, women are users of a whole series of substances that are
mind-altering. Women who use addictive substances are viewed as
either out of control, in need of control or both. Women who
'abuse' food are seen in a similar light.

Yet reflecting on the context of traditional discussions in the
addiction field one discovers that the terms 'addiction' or 'drug use'
do not mirror adequately women's somewhat problematic relationship to substances, regardless of whether or not they may be mind-
altering. This viewpoint is particularly important when we examine
women's relationship to food.

Chapter 1 noted that substance use is a gender-illuminating notion, enabling one to see more clearly women's dependence on food as an important theoretical concern within the addiction field. In that prior context, we saw how, for women, the notion of substance use, which implies varying levels of dependency on a variety of substances, can be linked with a general, feminist issue: dependency.

At this stage in the text we are aware that women rather than men appear to be prime casualties of the 'system of dependence' that is society. In this light, women who use substances, become depressed or 'go mad' can be seen as the victims of a system which encourages their psychological, emotional, physical, social and economic dependence on men. Ironically the above 'conditions' have a tendency to make women even more dependent upon a patriarchal health care system with an implicit medical ideology oppressive to women.

This chapter will examine a series of related issues which place women's 'dependence' upon food within a feminist perspective. These issues include the politics of global food consumption; the politicisation of women's bodies; food addiction as substance misuse; images of the ideal female body; women's flesh and the female body and a feminist view on the politics of dieting.

The politics of global food consumption

Most of us have very little if any recollection of our births. Nevertheless we are aware that immediately after our birth food became a major concern, not only for ourselves but also for our mothers. As Orbach (1978, p. 22) suggests, 'Women experience particular pressure over food and eating. After birth . . . breast or bottle becomes a major issue.'

On a global scale, women produce at least half of the world's output of food, mostly in poor, agricultural countries where they grow, harvest and prepare most of the food consumed by their families. In Africa they perform 60 to 80 per cent of agricultural work (Seager and Olson, 1986, p. 14). In western societies in particular, women do a large amount of the shopping for food

(Osman, 1983, p. 30). All of this suggests that women have a special relationship to food, regardless of whether or not they and their families have enough to live on or whether or not they have food in abundance.

Unlike drugs, food is a physical necessity for survival. Food is a basic source of energy and life. Humans must eat. These fundamental realities should be made explicit in feminist discussions on women and food, yet it is perhaps surprising that, in the relevant literature, there is an almost total absence of any discussion about the links between the feminisation of poverty, food shortages and starvation on a worldwide scale. The implication is that most work written by feminists in this area may reflect the needs and concerns of a privileged group of women: white, middle-class western women. That this group of women is confronted with an abundance of food in its societies, that these societies are fundamentally consumer cultures characterised by waste, and that the notions of waste and fat are relatively modern conceptions, developed alongside capital accumulation, should perhaps become more evident in discussions on women and food. Most importantly, that this group of women emerges from societies which not only control the world's food markets but also have created the notion of 'food addiction' should not be surprising.

Some women in developing countries are starving and unable to consider food as a reliable commodity. In some countries, to consider food as a basic resource is becoming increasingly difficult. On the other hand, the multi-million dollar 'fat industry', with its slimming products and diet organisations, finds its annual profits swelling as new global markets are developed. Weight Watchers (which began in the United States in 1961 and in Great Britain in 1967), Diet Kitchen, Diet Workshop, TOPS (Take Off Pounds Sensibly) and Overeaters Anonymous exist to exploit these ever-expanding markets. What one witnesses here is the gross economic inequalities existing between developed and developing countries. Behind these inequalities is the division between food consumption as a measure of affluence and food consumption as a matter of necessity. Within the context of the political economy of survival it has been suggested that the 'fat cats' in western nations characterised by the 'politics of greed' dominate almost totally the food distribution chain (*New Internationalist*, 1988).

In this context one should be aware that food, like health, power, wealth and privilege (Turner, 1987, p. 83) can be treated as a resource. The fact that this resource can be overconsumed through abundance, while being scarce in the poor countries of the world, may indicate a certain level of greed in developed countries. While greed or financial self-interest may be endemic in some forms of western capitalism, it can be seen as the 'very engine of social progress' (Brazier, 1988, p. 5). Within this view, monetary values are placed higher than human ones. As the 'fat industry', linked with the global food industry, extends, 'diet foods' are seen increasingly as a resource for those in affluent countries who have misused normal food. This is somewhat confusing given that normal food is no longer viewed as the only *real* resource in the area of food consumption.

Additionally one should also be aware that the food industry's distribution of surplus, unpopular or less nutritious normal food is less than responsible. Often large multinational food companies gain entry into highly lucrative markets by disposing of certain food products in the third world. This can be seen most clearly in the case of the baby milk scandal, involving the somewhat assertive marketing strategies of Nestlé, one of the largest food multinationals in the world. While free samples of baby milk were given to hospitals in Africa, mothers were encouraged to bottle-feed rather than breast-feed. In a feminist context it is perhaps not surprising that breast milk, the only food which is produced by the human body, specifically the female human body, should have been chosen as needing an artificial competitor, factory-produced milk. Breast milk is unprofitable and, furthermore, when a substitute is provided for it, the key role of women and women's bodies in the nurturing process is devalued and undermined.

The consequences of the baby bottle milk scandal were disastrous, given that these women had neither the money nor the sanitary facilities to bottle-feed on a regular, safe basis. While malnutrition, disease and death resulted, third-world women were encouraged to give up a safer, free and healthier means of feeding their babies. Women's bodies thus become subservient to market forces particularly if they live in a developing country where they have little influence and less control than if they lived in the developed world.

Whether women are encouraged to eat 'diet food' or to bottle-feed their babies, the female body is subjected to control and management. Large multinational food companies, based in affluent countries, have influence and continual surveillance over the distribution of food on a global scale. In effect, an international, hierarchical food chain is set up, establishing a powerful hold on the body, creating deeper divisions between developed and developing countries. While malnutrition and poverty reach epidemic proportions in various third-world countries, addiction to normal food or 'diet food' become widespread as millions of prosperous individuals compete with each other for more wealth and status. Within this view, women have more to lose than men both psychologically and economically. Women are seen to have a special relationship to food. But to understand this relationship one needs to explore the 'politicisation' of women's bodies and to see how this complex process affects women.

The politicisation of women's bodies

It has been argued that 'the body is directly involved in the political field . . . and becomes a useful force only if it is both a productive body and a subjected body' (Foucault, 1977, p. 26). Women more than men may experience themselves as 'subjected bodies'. This is because women's bodies more than men's bodies tend to be subordinated by violence and patriarchal ideology. The implication here is that, as a result of these 'instruments' of subjection, women's bodies are less directly involved in the political field. Yet, as Foucault points out, subjection of a 'physical order' may also be direct *without* involving violence. Given this insight, women's problematic relationship to food (food addiction) in developed countries may be an important, if not invisible, way of subjugating women's bodies. As Zweben (1987, p. 181) rightly asks: 'What does it mean that contemporary society, which is bombarded with diverse images of abundance, fosters a thinner and thinner ideal for women?'

In this context Orbach (1987, p. 4) contends that in contemporary society food and body-image issues can be seen as the language of women's inner experience. These issues need to be taken into the realm of women's psychological and social existence. Furthermore women should begin to assert their bodies as they *are* rather than as they should be. It is only when women recognise and make visible the very materiality of food as an instrument and vector of power on a global scale that they will be able to uncover and indeed liberate their subjected bodies as well as their inner experiences.

That there exists the need for women to assert their bodies as they 'are' reveals the inexorable link between food, diet and social power. That food and obsession with the body tends to dominate some if not many aspects of women's emotional and psychological lives may indicate that the politicisation of a woman's body may imply the politicisation of her 'soul'. For example, a woman's obsessions, fostering deep divisions between her spirit and her body, become effective tools to further subject her body to an image of who 'she should be'. While the misuse of a necessity (here food) by some women is indicative of economic and political abuse, it could be argued that this sort of misuse is part and parcel of the struggle for women's liberation: in order to liberate one's self as a subjected body, one needs to enter into the discourse on the politicisation of the body, bodily management and regulation. Women need to uncover the variety of tools and methods of power used over the body. Women need to expose how they, in particular, are caught up in a system of bodily subjection. Finally women need to break the link between food and the fetishisation of women's bodies.

It is quite interesting to note that for some women, food (Dickenson, 1983), like men (Delphy, 1984) is perceived as an enemy. In the former case, women's daily sustenance is viewed as a deadly foe, while in the latter case, women's traditional sexual partners in a heterosexist society are viewed as their main adversaries. On the one hand, food, a relatively non-threatening, inactive substance takes on a sinister, active quality; on the other, men as a social group become opponents in the 'gender war'. This discussion is primarily concerned with the former conception, food as an enemy; there are enormous political pitfalls with the latter conception. Yet if one takes a feminist stance, along with Ramaza-noglu (1989), one is able to assume that existing relations between the sexes in which women are subordinated to men are unsatisfac-tory and ought to be changed. Given that assumption, with any feminist issue such as women and food, one needs to uncover the ways in which any gendered system of dependence and domination is reproduced and can be challenged.

Food 'addiction' as substance misuse

In the previous discussion we have seen how the politicisation of women's bodies subjects women and uses the materiality of food as a vector of power. For all human beings, we *are* our bodies. One's relationship to the world is mediated through one's body. In addition eating, feeding and all the cultural and social rituals associated with these processes are important ways of validating and nurturing one's body and one's identity. For the majority of women, feeding others is viewed as a primary social role. The contradiction is that, for some women, particularly those in affluent societies, their relationship to food becomes problematic. More importantly this relationship may in which become a principal way in which the problem of their female being comes to expression in women's lives (Chernin, 1985). As Lawrence (1987, p. 12) contends, 'eating disorders for us are not merely troublesome symptoms which need to be eradicated'. Neither are they primarily 'forms of self-addiction' (Huseman, Madison, Pearson, Leuschen, 1990). They go much deeper than the level of symptom and addiction.

In this context, Boskind-White (1981, p. 54) suggests that obesity, anorexia and bulimia are complicated eating disorders: 'the latter two are twin sisters, with obesity viewed as the evil stepsister'. The above ideas demonstrate that for women there is a distinct though sometimes hidden connection between eating, feeding and the struggle for identity.

A discussion of eating as a form of substance misuse becomes complicated when this connection is considered more closely. There is a need to understand how women's problematic relationship with food is perceived by experts who define and treat the problem as well as by the women who experience the problem. In this context, three basic questions will be asked to develop our understanding: (1) why is there such a concept as food addiction; (2) what does it represent; and (3) what is the relationship between food addiction and drug addiction as forms of substance misuse?

Firstly, the concept, 'food addiction', covers all forms of what the experts term 'eating disorders' (that is, bulimia, anorexia and compulsive eating) whether these disorders are characterised by ingesting or expelling food. While the author has shied away from using the term 'addiction' in her theoretical work, she has demonstrated the usefulness of the concept 'substance use' as a gender-illuminating notion. On the other hand, in this discussion, the author will employ the term 'food addiction' to demonstrate how the dual notions of dependence ('of the subordinate thing kind' and 'of the addiction kind') come into play with regard to women's relationship to, their use and their misuse of food. Whether or not a woman with a food problem gains or loses weight, starves, overeats or vomits should not be seen as the key issue. Rather one should direct concern towards the way women's obsession with food is linked with their obsession with their bodies.

It is clear from the literature in this area that 'the variety of disordered eating patterns observed clinically bears little clear relationship to weight' (Wooley and Wooley, 1981, p. 43). This implies that it is on perceived body size rather than actual body weight that women 'food addicts' tend to 'fixate'.

Secondly, from previous discussions in this chapter, we have seen that food as a vector of power has been consistently used as a material and natural 'instrument' through which women are addressed. While women are more often than not casualties of a system of dependence, food is a very powerful, if not the most primitive, means for women to respond to this system. Whether or not women overeat, 'binge' eat or refuse to eat, the issue of dependency appears to be a central concern.

Women may eat to alleviate 'dependence on the judgement of male society as a basis for self-esteem' (Boskind-Lodahl, 1976). They may eat to respond to stress as a substitute gratification when other areas of life provide few satisfactions (Hamburger, 1951). Regardless of the complex reasons, women addicted to food or abusing food 'defy' their acceptable female role. In a real sense, they are taking extreme control over their own food intake. Whether or not their eating habits are seen as out of control (through over-eating, binging and/or vomiting) or too controlling (through dieting and/or starving themselves), these women are saying a distinct 'no' to what is perceived as women's normal relationship to food. Ultimately their message is: 'We will eat what we want, when we want and as much or as little as we want.'

Lastly it should not be surprising that food addiction and drug addiction as forms of substance misuse are emblematic of a woman's response to an oppressive social system. For example, as Orbach (1987, p. 29) claims, 'in the most tortuous denial of need and dependency and the most persistent and insistent expression of independence, women with anorexia live out the contrariness of contemporary cultural dictates'. One could add that *all* women who experience a problematic relationship with substances are asserting an independence while defying a system of dependence. Yet food, unlike drugs, cannot be given up completely.

On a deeper level, Kim Chernin (1981, p. 2) contends that for women 'the body holds meaning'. A woman seen to be abusing her body through food or other substances may be expressing the fact that she feels uncomfortable being female in this culture. However, as the reader is aware, substance misuse, whether it is food-related or drugs-related, may have serious consequences for the female user. Therefore women caught in this quandary between defiance and misuse need hope. That women need to have control over their own bodies and what goes into these bodies is essential. Their control offers a direct challenge to traditional practices which select women as vessels of abuse, violence, degradation, subordination and restriction.

Images of the 'ideal' female body

The implication in the previous discussions is that any woman who has a problem with food will also have a problem with her body. If food is the instrument through which a woman is addressed, her body is the medium through which female meaning, subjectivity, materiality and power are dealt with. If a woman is obsessed with the size of her body, she is inevitably plagued by the size of her appetite for food. By establishing a closer link between women's obsession with food and women's obsession with her body, one is establishing a link between women's eating and women's struggle for identity. More often than not this struggle permeates a woman's entire life.

Obsession with one's body usual means that one is desperately concerned to conform to the idealised feminine form which is fat-free, small and relatively weak. As Brownmiller (1984, p. 17) suggests:

> Fleshiness is problematic to the present-day feminine illusion, for while fat creates the celebrated dimorphic curves of womanhood, it is also the

agent of massiveness and bulk, properties readily associated with masculine solidity and power.

Additionally small is beautiful for women. As Brown (1987) suggests, when women are small they occupy less space, are less visible and utilise less resources. She also notes that, while women are valued culturally by their adherence to this rule, the precise dimensions of correct smallness have varied across time according to the whims of various social control agents (that is, men): patriarchal standards of 'fat' and 'thin' can be highly erratic and variable.

Diamond (1985, p. 50) asserts that in contemporary society 'advertising for beauty preparations, fashion, diet and health products all construct the ideal as the "slim female body" and . . . that conceptions of femininity are intertwined with these notions of the natural and health'. However there is a discrepancy. There exists an irresolvable tension between women's inner feelings about themselves as women and their own identities as women: a problem arises between a woman's outer experiences of her body and society's expectation of what she is to do with her body. A discussion of women's conflicting experience of becoming pregnant and the reality of becoming mothers should help to clarify these ideas.

For example, for all women, heterosexual, bisexual or lesbian, motherhood is seen as the epitome of womanhood. But the 'high pedestal–low status' mentality which surrounds motherhood means that mothers are given little status and few facilities to ease or enrich their lives (Sharpe, 1984, p. 42); their hopes of self-fulfilment are slim. To become a mother, a woman obviously needs to become pregnant. Regardless of how she becomes pregnant, a woman will inevitably develop an awareness that to be fully pregnant is to become 'fat'. It is to have a roundness which is perceived as being a 'natural' part of the process of child bearing. This is perhaps the only time in a woman's life when she knows at a deep level that to be fat, pregnant and round is to be a 'good' woman. In a real sense, to be round is to be female. Yet in a society which devalues women the image of women as life-giving can be deeply threatening. Confirming this point, Kelly (1983, p. 20) says:

> Round is female. Round females are the visual symbols of strength, love, of life-giving. When you start getting in touch with the fact that being round and being big is very female, then you begin to understand why

men have asked us to go away. They want us to be little, smaller than they are.

Whether or not women are pregnant, women do experience at times a feeling of emptiness, a 'lack of self' and an estrangement from the 'original' woman – 'the woman who searches for and claims her relational origins with her vital Self and with other women' (Raymond, 1986, p. 5). In order to gain a sense of self-esteem, to find self-love and ultimately to be in touch with the 'original' woman, women need to assert the power and abundance of the feminine. As Chernin (1981, p. 101) suggests, women should seek to widen their frame of reference, to be expansive, to enlarge their views, to acquire weight and to fill out, rather than to reduce themselves, to become small, to narrow themselves, to become lightweight or to belittle themselves, as is the practice in standard weight-watching groups.

If women expand themselves and, therefore, establish a link with the 'original' woman, they are challenging a culture that is profoundly divided within itself. They begin to probe beneath the surface of a society which divides the apparent nature of woman from the apparent nature of man. Women's alienation from their natural source of female power and energy becomes visible in this process. Objectively this probing is a positive step, exposing the limitations imposed on women's emotional and sexual life.

Women's flesh and the female body

As suggested earlier, if a woman is obsessed with her body size and her appetite for food, she may also be obsessed with the size of her sexual appetite. In this context, it is interesting to note that nineteenth-century physicians regarded anorexia as one of the manifold forms of hysteria which not only had a central role in psychiatric discourse but also in definitions of femininity and female sexuality (Showalter, 1985, p. 129). While hysteria is derived from the Greek word, 'hystera', meaning womb, it became a word intrinsically linked with extremes of emotionality. That the womb is the seat of emotions and that women are seen to be more emotional than men (Griffin, 1978, p. 13) implies that hysteria is linked intrinsically with what it means to be a woman. When the body troubles women it may be because this body needs feeding. On the other hand, this body is filled with urges and appetites that 'we cannot control and are not able to transcend' (Chernin, 1981, p. 56).

Given that Eve, the archetypical woman, is viewed as flesh, all women can be seen as flesh. While their 'beauty is a lure . . . their bodies are made for seduction' (Griffin, 1978, p. 83). Whether these ideas are denied or accepted, the revelation of women's flesh in society is surrounded by myths and deception. Griffin (1981, p. 30) contends that the intensified mythology developed around women's bodies has had dramatic effects:

> We believe a woman is naturally modest, ashamed of her own body, afraid by nature to reveal her flesh. And on the other hand we believe the sight of her flesh has a transformative effect on the mind of a man . . . For if a woman by her beauty can make a man into a rapist, she can also transform him in other ways. Her overwhelming seductive powers can lead him into the world of the flesh and the devil.

Whether or not women are too large (whether physically or otherwise), women are flesh and women's flesh is more often than not perceived as evil. It is not surprising that feeding/eating is a problematic area for many women, when women's appetite for food is linked to women's appetite for sex. Both appetites remind women of their bodies. More specifically, through their 'passion' for both food and sex, women remind themselves that their flesh exists not for themselves but for the Other, man.

Fursland (1987, p. 16) suggests that women have felt guilty with regard to sexual matters for many years, a process culminating in nineteenth-century Victorian values. But, she adds, 'food is replacing sex as the focus of guilt in women's lives'. In a different light, a woman wishing to control her hungers and urges 'may be expressing the fact that she has been taught to regard her emotional life, her passions and "appetites" as dangerous, requiring control and careful monitoring' (Chernin, 1981, p. 2). While her flesh is evil, her hungers are harmful to herself and society.

In a discussion of the complex causes which transformed diet in the late nineteenth century into a secular science for the rationalisation of the body, Turner (1987, pp. 26–7) demonstrates how, for contemporary consumer culture, the thin body is the symbol of youthfulness, activity and health. Turner contends that, while religious, monastic practices of earlier centuries focused on management of the inner body, contemporary, secular consumerism is concerned with a discipline of the surfaces of the body. With regard to this discipline, the self is enhanced and displayed by the absence of flesh. Therefore to be fat is not only to be out of control but also to lack a 'consumer asceticism'.

While Turner is sympathetic to a feminist perspective and includes a discussion of the discourse of bodily management and regulation with regard to women's bodies, he takes a somewhat uncritical view of flesh and more specifically women's materiality *vis à vis* men's. For Turner, the obese woman is a woman out of control because the unrestrained body is 'indicative of moral laxity' (p. 108). Extending Turner's argument one could say that, regardless of a woman's body weight and her excessive appetite for food, women more than men are viewed as having greater tendencies to moral laxity *by the very fact* that they are women. Common perceptions of women's flesh sets up this discontinuity. Therefore all women, whether they are fat or thin lack 'consumer asceticism'. Women experience this lack primarily because a women's sense of being 'in the flesh' is placed, consciously or not, in opposition to men's sense of being in the whole corporeal world.

Women's perception of their bodies, their body images and their knowledge of the oppressive values inherent in a consumer society generate an awareness that success in their female role relates to the 'normal', male-defined, physical image which traditional (that is, male-defined) women create and project. In effect women experience their own bodies, their flesh as both commodities and objects. Orbach (1986, p. 104) illustrates this point quite clearly:

> Not only is it the case that women's sphere of activity has frequently been directed into consumerism, but that there is a complex relationship between women's bodies and the fact that their bodies are so very much both commodity and object for them in the world. The world allows women to enter into a circumscribed way, to occupy particular spaces.

Women's space in the world is delineated and controlled. Any woman's body and flesh, occupying a specific space in the material world, can be viewed as risky, requiring management and careful supervision. In this context, it is interesting to note that 'figure control is one of the few forms of control most women are allowed to exercise' (Mayer, 1983, p. 3).

In a society that sees women as a commodity and the object of men's sexual desires, thin women as opposed to fat women have a higher selling power. This process sets up a unique hierarchy in which thin is privileged. Thin is a more highly valued state of fleshiness than fat. The most damaging effect of this hierarchy is that a wedge is driven between fat women and thin women. Thin women as opposed to fat women are seen as more sexually attractive, more conforming to male images of the female body and generally more feminine.

Given this dilemma, a women-oriented view questions not only contemporary consumerist values, making women commodities and sexual objects, but also literature which may unwittingly continue deep divisions between women on the basis of body size. In an article on the notion of thin as a feminist issue, Diamond (1985, p. 63) is very clear on this point:

> A feminist construction should tend toward diversity, with space being made for a new array of possibilities for bodily imagery, definitions of identity, women's multiple pleasures: alternatives that only a collective movement can create.

The concluding section of this chapter will examine some of the alternatives that have been created by women in their struggle with new concerns vital for changing conceptions of women's bodies. There is a need to develop new conceptual alternatives that will be more sensitive to women. Furthermore this sensitivity implies unearthing a hidden need: to view desire and pleasure as a means of transforming women's political arena.

A feminist view of the 'politics' of dieting

In recent years, women attempting to achieve the 'ideal' female body size have either been organised or have organised themselves in self-help groups concerned with dieting and overeating. Not only is it 'good' to be slim but also it is 'good' to be seen to be fit and healthy. For many women an interest in health and fitness has turned into 'the cult of the body' (Mitchell, 1987, p. 156). This distinct preference for a healthy type of body represents what has been referred to as 'healthism' (Zola, 1991), implying a level of alienation.

Objectively diet organisations and self-help groups such as Weight Watchers and Overeaters Anonymous exist to help their members (the majority being women) to reduce their fat by reducing their food intake. This process usually requires that members buy 'special diet foods', expanding the markets of the 'diet industry', attend special groups to talk about ways of overcoming their dependence upon food and, ultimately, sort out their problems with others who share them. In reality, these groups uphold conventional male images of the acceptable woman and are implicitly male-defined.

When *Fat is a Feminist Issue* was first published in 1978, Susie Orbach related her experiences of women-only self-help groups, dealing specifically with body image, helping women to rethink many previously held assumptions about women's eating habits. In effect these self-help groups have mounted a challenge to the food industry's, specifically the diet industry's, subtle control over women's bodies. While Noble (1987, p. 134) has outlined in detail the strengths and weaknesses of these feminist self-help groups as a growing movement, she contends that 'self-help is a powerful and healing process that has helped thousands of women to help themselves and change their lives for the better'.

The overall dynamics of feminist self-help groups has been liberating and enriching for women (Ernst and Goodison, 1981) and a feminist would be hard-pressed to deny the generative effect of consciousness raising, a powerful dynamic within these groups. Yet it has been argued that the 'fat is a feminist issue' philosophy is anti-diet; it is a philosophy set up in opposition to the body regime of diets, exercise and self-control and it speaks in similar terms as the conventional diet philosophy, foisted upon all women (Diamond, 1985).

From the perspective of fat women's liberation, Dickenson (1983, p. 42) criticises the 'fat is a feminist issue' philosophy as a case of victim blaming ('Thinness is best, it is a woman's duty to try for it, and therefore it is her fault if she fails.'). Dickenson also takes issue with any feminist analysis which ignores the economic roots of fat (that is to say, money and food are intertwined) or excludes women of colour and poor women. In a similar vein, Kowalski (1984,

p. 213) contends that the stereotypes which are attached to fat women are 'lies':

> We have all swallowed the myths put out by the medical 'experts' – even those of us who are sceptical and even downright disbelieving . . . The oppression of fat wimmin is based on looks and looks only. Yet everyone has their own particular pet theory as to why we should lose weight – the fact is that we can't – fat wimmin are biologically fat – I'm a fat woman and I do know what I'm talking about!

For the fat woman liberationist, a deep hostility to fat is seen to exist in society. Fat is perceived as 'dangerous' and 'unhealthy' (Bovery, 1989). In reality hatred of fat stems from hatred of women. Furthermore orthodox beauty images tend to be informed by race, sex and class. It could be argued further in this context that hatred of fat stems from hatred of the female, the 'mother' and anything or any person that is seen to be weak.

From a feminist perspective, based on her clinical experience with women, Brown (1987, p. 297) asserts that women are valued only when they adhere unfailingly to the following four rules: (1) small is beautiful; (2) weakness of the body is valued; (3) women are forbidden to nurture themselves in a straightforward or ego syntonic manner; and (4) women are forbidden to act powerfully in overt ways.

The implication of Brown's assertions is that women are devalued and often stigmatised for their visibility, their solidity and their 'substance'. The contradiction is that, as more women become economically, politically and socially visible and substantial in a women-devaluing society, the more women will find that their female space is limited both psychologically and domestically. Female space tends to be defined by traditional male customs, images and attitudes. As this space is defined in the home, 'liberating' technological innovations bind women to domesticity more closely than ever (Murcott, 1983). When this process unfolds, women become further removed from their women selves.

For women devalued for their substance, defining their own space, their own flesh, their own sexualities and their own relationships to their bodies may be a liberating experience. It was suggested earlier that women experiencing problems with food and, in turn, their bodies need to find their original Female Selves:

the 'original woman'. In this search they learn to transform traditional male concepts of desire and pleasure, identified as women's own 'pure lust for metamorphosis' (Daly, 1984). In other words, as women search for their real selves, they develop a deep appetite for psychic transformation. While some readers may criticise these ideas as obtuse or inaccessible, this type of approach establishes the need for the 'revalorization of feminine elements and qualities' (French, 1984, p. 484) – women's experience becomes important and revalued. This type of framework also establishes a new women-centred way of observing and criticising outdated modes of thinking about woman, her body and her social space. This process helps to generate an appetite for change, essential for social transformation. Therefore, whether as fat women or thin women, women attempt to become women of substance for themselves.

Let us look more closely at the significance of these ideas in the context of the above discussions. For any woman, her 'appetite' or lust has been defined as 'pure Passion: unadulterated, absolute, simple, sheer striving for abundance of be-ing' (Daly, 1988, p. 89). This appetite implies that women involve themselves in a process in which they choose to escape being devalued and follow their 'heart's deepest desire'. If women involve themselves in this process, they experience deep psychic changes or metamorphosis. These deep changes reflect 'changes of physical/spiritual form or substance' (Daly, 1988, p. 81). In the light of Daly's comments, it could be argued that as women begin to take positive steps towards change, they experience a change of 'substance', whether on a physical or a spiritual level.

As this change occurs, primary concerns in the debates about women's food addiction and body image are rethought and, in turn, redirected towards fundamental questions: how do women shift the shape of being, thinking and imagining in an outdated world structured by the inequalities of gender, race and class? How do women go about changing the damaging images imposed on them regarding their bodies, their 'wicked flesh', their 'moral laxity' and their 'lack of consumer asceticism'? And how do women transform traditional female images of themselves into sources of enchantment with their real female selves?

In this field of study there is an urgent need to transform the negative into the positive. Carving out paths of understanding that can no longer be reached by conventional means may be necessary. For instance, the final goal is to value oneself as a woman. This movement signifies a new experience for women substance users as they revalue and reclaim themselves and their bodies. This distinct process is a feminist process, symbolising 'experience of and through emotion charged with thought', rather than thought charged with emotion (French, 1985, p. 490). By charging emotions with thought, women are able better to transform for themselves the 'cult of the body' into the cult of women of substance. As Daly (1984, p. 389) says: 'Like Sirens singing the call of the Strange, Be-Witching women rearrange the shape of our lives. We are Shape-shifters, in ontological dimensions.'

In conclusion, caught up in this ontological dimension, some women may feel the need to shift their bodily shapes, while others may not. However all women attempting to understand their relationship to food and ultimately their bodies could benefit by viewing themselves as 'shape-shifters'. The crucial idea is that traditional images of women's bodies need to change into images reflective of women's 'substance', their strength and their integrity.

7

A feminist response to substance abuse

One can't really be a revolutionary without being cognizant of the need to link up with forces all over the world battling with imperialism . . . Led by women, the fight for the liberation of women must be embraced by men as well . . . Black women constitute the most oppressed sector of society. (Angela Davis, 'Prison Interviews' in A. Y. Davis, R. Magee, the Soledad Brothers and other political prisoners (1971), *If They Come in the Morning*)

Introduction

Thus far, we have looked at a variety of substances used by women: alcohol, minor tranquillisers, heroin, tobacco and food. Challenging traditional notions of addiction, we have seen how dependency on substances reflects in many ways women's social positioning, specifically her own dependency 'of a subordinate thing kind'. A structural, feminist analysis which should be useful to women users, clinicians and researchers alike has been offered. It has been consistently suggested that we need to establish a broad base of understanding and knowledge in this area of concern in order to move on to a real meeting of women substance users' needs. It is hoped that the discussions in the previous chapters have helped the reader to generate an awareness of the usefulness as well as the need for a feminist perspective in the field of substance use.

This chapter will examine the potential for effective social action *vis-à-vis* women substance users. The basic assumption is that women's praxis, while existing in seed form, should be nurtured, encouraged and developed in the field. Before this process is able to unfold, all who are concerned with the issue of women and substance use should have a clear understanding of the answers to the following *fundamental* questions.

With special reference to women, how has substance use been defined? From which historical context does the politics of women's substance use emerge? What models for intervention or change exist in the substance use field? Within these models, where do women fit in and is there any room for women's political mobilisation? What types of feminist strategies are needed both collectively and individually for women substance users to achieve increased visibility and effectiveness? These questions will be answered in the following discussions.

Defining substance use: 'individualisation' and 'positive addiction'

Before placing the women and substance use issue in a political context we need to have an overview of the general models of addiction as well as the kinds of ideas that already exist on women and addiction. Furthermore we need to asses whether or not these models and ideas can be used constructively in the process of social transformation. Real social change demands effective social action, based on definitions of addiction which enable the generation of a collective consciousness for women. At the heart of this consciousness and feminist action is a structural critique of women's position within a dependence-producing society.

Reflecting on their work involvement with chemically dependent women, Peluso and Peluso (1988) discuss how these women abide in fundamentally different cultures from men and face challenges that are compounded by the fact that they are women. With an awareness of women's 'patterns of experience', the authors contend that the male-oriented disease model of addiction has been a subtle way of blocking women out of the picture all together. For the Pelusos, social factors rather than genetic or biological factors explain the pattern of experiences for the chemically dependent woman:

> The majority of chemically dependent women cite difficult life events as precipitating factors in their drug use. Typically, a woman uses chemicals

to reduce stress and to cope with her life, and to anaesthetize her painful, negative feelings. If we view the chemically dependent woman as a victim of the very same disease that strikes men, we ignore the unique situational stresses and cultural pressures that impact her – and all women. (p. 184)

What is of interest here is that these authors accept the disease model for men but not for women. Chemical dependence is seen to be 'more social' for women than for men who experience a greater predisposition to a 'real' disease (that is, addiction) with indications of a genetic factor. The key is that for women addicts their *feelings* about their social and political circumstances interface with the physical processes of addiction. Therefore any change is directed towards individual women rather than the overall society which structures women's circumstances or predisposes them as a group to addiction and dependency. While 'feeling different' may be an important part of the reality of women substance users, this notion appears to take priority over fundamental notions, such as women's praxis or collective consciousness. An emphasis on individual feelings rather than collective human rights thwarts the development of a critical analysis in this area. While women's feelings are relatively clear, their real social needs remains invisible.

In this type of model, regardless of whether the emphasis is on personal factors or social factors, addiction is individualised and in turn depoliticised. The individual woman or man is the focus and indeed locus of change. Interestingly enough, this sort of work extends the notion of addiction to include love, relationships and life itself, as we will see later in the discussion. As a result those truly sensitive to and accepting of this addiction approach become 'superior' individuals, moving from control of the body to discipline of the mind. More importantly the body is subordinated not only to bodily regulation but also to a sort of spiritual awakening. The Pelusos say (1988, p. 197): 'Every recovering woman we spoke with in the course of writing this book had experienced a spiritual awakening, a belief in god, or a higher power, and started living with hope.'

Perhaps at this stage in our discussion it would be worthwhile to look more closely at other work which 'individualises' addiction. Bradshaw (1988, p. viii) sees addiction as 'toxic shame', the feeling which 'destroys the functioning of our authentic selves'. While personal mortification is linked up with addiction, the individual wanting to break from this 'habit' is ultimately free to move on to 'habitual' fellowship with others coping in a more acceptable way with their 'shame'. In a similar vein, Stewart (1984) views all addictions as 'love disorders'. The disordered lover is an addict and all addicts 'need to move from the lone self, caught up in ego problems, to the interaction of person with person – from self-will to good will, from control to discipline' (p.x).

Another author (Norwood, 1986, p. 205) looks at women who love too much and argues that these women are afflicted with 'a disease process' and are in 'the grip of a pattern over which they have lost control'. The cause of this 'disease' is that they emerge from dysfunctional homes in which their emotional needs are unmet. In this model, Norwood's 'women who love enough' are immersed in positive affirmations, which help them to enjoy perfect peace and well-being and guide them to their highest happiness and fulfilment. They are not only disciplined and full of good will (building a circle of well friends) but also conformist and recovered from their 'dysfunctional' upbringing.

While women who love too much use men as their 'drug of escape', it could be argued that women who love enough use their positivity as a 'drug of involvement'. They become addicted to being positive and thus deny negative emotions such as anger and rage which have the potential to be healing for many, if not all women. In effect, 'women who love enough' become addicted to being what society expects of all women: compliant, conformist, always ready to love with a smile, wanting to please and never angry.

'Positive addiction' (PA) has been identified as a necessary part of life and Glasser (1976) offers six steps to PA in order to fulfil one's daily fix or need for a beneficial obsession. The six criteria are that an activity be non-competitive, easy to perform, solitary, valuable (mentally, physically or spiritually) to the person, subjectively measured and carried out without criticising oneself. In this model, meditators and runners represent the two largest categories of those in a PA state.

As we can see these authors attempt to shift the addiction debate to a new moral discourse, positive addiction. Regulation of habits and collective interaction are the cure, replacing the traditional need for unauthentic, shameful selves to control their unrestrained bodies. Shared or collective discipline of the mind governs moral laxity and ensures spiritual consciousness and ultimately, consensus. Any addiction reflecting this state of awareness ensures individual growth. Positive addiction is OK, negative addiction is not OK and only the individual is able to *feel* the difference.

Feeling the difference: process addiction and substance addiction

In this context, Schaef and Fassel (1988, p. 58) contend that anything can be used addictively (whether they be processes or substances) because the 'purpose of an addiction is to put a buffer between ourselves and our awareness or feelings'. For these authors substance addictions are ingestive, while process addiction 'refers to a series of activities or interactions that hook a person or on which a person becomes dependent' (sex, work, money, religion and so on) (p. 58). All addictions numb individuals so that 'we are out of touch with what we know and what we *feel*' (p. 58). The contention is that through addiction one blocks out an awareness of other aspects of one's life, needed for self-discovery and spiritual recovery. Again we see that discipline of the mind governs moral negligence and restores a sort of metaphysical order. Feelings are paramount, while the body is merely a vehicle for the displacement of feelings, not the enactment of psychological 'hooks'.

Focusing specifically on substance addiction, other authors (Brown, Manderson, O'Callaghan and Thompson, 1986) argue that all individuals need their 'daily fix of drugs' which have a symbolic significance in society. While legal drugs are regarded as totems, illegal drugs are viewed as taboo and never the twain shall meet – that is, unless the symbols change, and sometimes they do. For example, contrast the popular usage of opium in the mid to late nineteenth century, documented by Berridge and Edwards (1981), with today's classification of opium as a 'dangerous drug'. In the 'totem and taboo model', drug use is individualised but social discipline regulates what *symbolises* moral negligence at any given historical moment. In other words permissiveness is governed by social forces rather than by individual needs (Dorn, 1980).

From the above there is little evidence of a critical, social model of addiction. As regards women, we are left with the view that, if families were functional, women would not experience 'dependence of the addiction thing kind'. This view is a subtle case of victim blaming: if mothers were really good mothers, there families would not be dysfunctional. In addition, there is little room to look critically at the way the concept of a functional family may relate directly to 'dependence of the subordinate thing kind'.

While it is useful to see that the 'patterns of experience' differ for men and women substance users, it is essential to know that within society, these patterns are produced historically by the sex–gender, race and class systems. Clearly we need a transformative shift in this field, a shift derived from the envelopment of a well-defined feminist epistemology, the basis for women's praxis.

Women's praxis and women's health: developing a feminist epistemology

The generation of a feminist awareness of the women and substance use issue has some identifiable roots in the women's health movement, based on the need for a collective social approach to the problems of women's ill health. While this movement emerges from the Women's Liberation Movement (WLM), it has consistently emphasised the need for women's self-help, women-centred health education, women-centred health care provision and campaigns about specific feminist health care issues. In this area women's praxis is focused on developing strategies which ensure women's physical as well as emotional well-being. Women's praxis envelops a strategic approach which aims to abolish any obstacles to the achievement of a more caring, humane approach to women's public health.

While individually focused medicine does not consider the social origins of many illnesses, the women's health movement has attempted to shift this focus to wider concerns. In this context, Thunhurst (1982, pp. 62–3) says:

> We are often blamed, implicitly or explicitly, for ill-health which has its origin in the social roles that we fill, or in our personal rejection of these roles. Women, in particular, have suffered from this . . . The individual is treated when attention ought to be directed towards the individual's social experience. The awareness that the social experience is producing ill health will normally indicate that the correct remedial action is social action.

Feminist social action in the health field is concerned with changing consciousness, providing health-related services and struggling to change established health institutions (Fruchter, Fatt, Booth and Leidel, 1977). It is also to do with educating ourselves to see that the control of our health and fertility is fundamental to the control of our lives (Boston Women's Health Collective (British edition), 1978). The implications here are that medicine, more than a servicing profession, is an institution of social control and that women need to understand their oppression at the hands of the medical profession before they can change it.

Reflecting on the origins of feminist health activism, Lesley Doyal (1983) outlines the historical stages of the British women's health movement and focuses on the concept of reproduction (both ideological and biological) as a useful one in explaining the relationship between women and medicine. She argues that on the ideological level, 'medical knowledge and practice are part of the means by which gender divisions in society are maintained' (p. 379). Medicine is deeply involved in the reproduction of a specific view of the intrinsic character of women. In effect medicine does not invent our social roles, it merely interprets them to women as biological destiny (Ehrenreich and English, 1974).

Clearly the relationship between women's bodies, biological reproduction and medicine is an oppressive one in which women lose out. While Doyal (1983) is aware that medicine plays a part in the overall reproduction of the relations of production, she also recognises the importance of biological reproduction:

> if social relations are to remain basically unchanged and capital accumulation is to be maximally facilitated, then some degree of social control has to be exercised over women's sexuality over who gives birth and under what conditions. (p. 379)

Doyal and Elston (1986, p. 202) argue that, within a feminist critique of medicine, women have generated political responses focused on four key areas of activity: 're-defining women as healthy; overcoming women's ignorance; attacking sexist beliefs and practices and seizing the means of reproduction for themselves'. In the light of the above and with special reference to the substance use field, it could be argued that the women and substance use issue has emerged and become visible more from within traditional self-help groups – Narcotics Anonymous (NA), Alcoholics Anonymous (AA), Adult Children of Alcoholics (ACOA), Overeaters Anonymous, Weight Watchers and so on – than from the WLM or specifically, the women's health movement. Although a feminist analysis of substance use exists in seed form in the WLM, a greater awareness of the dual notions of dependency needs to be generated in order to challenge the dominance of traditional self-help groups in this area. Given the lack of feminist awareness in the substance use field, it is fair to say that the areas of activity mentioned above remain underdeveloped, if not undeveloped.

The dominance of 'traditional' self-help groups: the clinical model

In order to establish a clear picture of the dominance of traditional self-help groups in the substance use field, we should look briefly at the general process of self-help, the dynamics of traditional self-help groups in the field of substance abuse and the specific impact that these groups have had on women.

Sketching the fundamentals of self-help groups for drug misuse, Einstein (1983, p. 560) suggests that self-help is not a homogeneous entity and that it is often assumed that self-help should be turned to as a last resort because the traditional forms of intervention have failed. While it is not appropriate in this discussion to review the existing literature on self-help, it is fitting to specify that two distinct historical models of self-help have been identified: the clinical model and the structural model (Pancoast, Parker and Froland, 1983). (For a sound review of the existing self-help literature, see Richardson and Goodman, 1983). Within the former, clinical model, self-help is a means by which individuals or small groups can deal with their own problems and survive in a world for which they are seen not to be ideally suited. On the other hand, self-help within the structural model is seen as a natural and healthy way for communities to organise themselves both for internal and social satisfaction and against loss of control and lack of social awareness.

It could be argued that those involved in the clinical model collude with society by accepting their victim role; they focus on individual enlightenment rather than group consciousness and make little, if any, attempt to question why in a society supposedly based on social welfare principles, they need to 'help themselves'. Alternatively it appears that those involved in the structural model of self-help reject victimisation, attempt to generate a collective awareness based on the notion of struggle and confirm that social well-being, based on the pleasurable effects of participating in a just, equal society, is a fundamental social need as well as a basic human right.

NA and AA are the two most visible, socially acceptable self-help groups for both men and women substance users. Different groups which focus on other addictions include Overeaters Anonymous, Emotions Anonymous, Sex and Love Addicts Anonymous, Al-Anon and Al-ATeen. Other self-help groups with a supposedly feminist sensitivity such as Women for Sobriety (Kirkpatrick, 1977) or ACOA (Woititz, 1983) uphold wholeheartedly the disease model, a model which we have seen is not conducive to political action in the substance use field.

While the worth of these types of self-help groups for many addicts or substance users must not be denied, it is suggested that these mixed settings do not provide the optimum environment for women of varying ages, sexual orientations, social classes and ethnic origins to empower themselves. Given that institutionalised forms of oppression, such as sexism and racism, tend to rear their ugly heads in such highly-charged and emotional settings, women and people of colour tend to lose out. Furthermore I would suggest that these sorts of self-help groups, based on the clinical model of self-help and focused on individual enlightenment, use individual and group disclosure rather than consciousness raising as an operating principle. While consciousness raising has been identified as a powerful dynamic of social change, particularly for women (Payne, 1973), any development of women's praxis in these settings is questionable.

While the male focus of AA has been recognised (Al-Anon Family Groups, 1973, p. 67), there has been little attempt within AA to look critically at or to question male dominance within the home. AA works towards not only 'restoring families to the good life' but also re-establishing the power of the 'head of the family', which is of course the man (AA, 1967, p. 190).

Talking out a problem (Robinson, 1979), rather than challenging social divisions which create these problems, is the *modus vivendi* for membership in these groups which tend to be dominated by white, middle-class men. Given this type of domination, NA, AA and other addiction self-help groups may be insensitive to the ways in which capital, patriarchy and race structure women's oppression and exploitation (Parmar, 1982). The development of both a feminist consciousness and an anti-racist stance appears as yet unattainable within these self-help groups.

NA, AA and other similar self-help groups tend to be politically sterile because they operate within the clinical model of self-help and can be insensitive to the needs of women and black people. In effect they do not attempt to redress the organisational imbalances, stifling a potential for social change.

Women's self-help and women's substance use: a structural model

Alongside the rise of the self-help groups identified above, the increased politicisation of the notion of self-help has emerged as a new social force, associated with the women's liberation movement (WLM), the civil rights movement, the gay liberation movement, the anti-poverty movement and the youth movement: all of which embody the structural concept of self-help.

As implied earlier in this chapter, the impact of self-help within the WLM has been felt primarily in areas of women's health such as childcare, reproductive rights, contraception and abortion. (See for example, Boston Women's Health Collective, 1971, 1978.) Since the mid-1970s there has been a proliferation of women's groups actively concerned with establishing more knowledge of and control over women's own bodies. As Hanmer (1985) suggests, initially 'control over our bodies' referred to biological reproduction and, in particular, abortion, while in recent years the implications of this slogan have been extended to the areas of sexuality and childcare. Through the WLM, a collective awareness of the need for control over one's body was generated and the issues of sex, gender and biological reproduction, traditionally private issues, were thrust into the public sphere.

Through self-help and consciousness raising, women involved in the WLM were able to create amongst themselves a renewed sense of solidarity and strength. The desired effect of consciousness raising was sisterhood and cohesive political action (Yates, 1975). 'Sisterhood was seen as powerful' (Morgan, 1970) and 'empowerment' became the 'buzz word' within the WLM. Although today the WLM movement does not attract the same level of media attention as in earlier years, many women of all age groups, all races, all sexual orientations, are active in a variety of areas and a plethora of women's issues.

The establishment of DAWN (Drugs, Alcohol and Woman Nationally) in 1976 by a group of feminists working in the area of substance abuse has had a significant impact in the area of women and substance abuse in Britain (McConville, 1983). Initially the work of DAWN focused on raising the consciousness of women workers, subjected to male clinicians or bosses, operating within the framework of outdated, sterile, sexist attitudes and practices. Since the establishment of DAWN (London) in February 1983, organisational attention has turned towards the generation of a feminist perspective on women and dependency as well as the establishment of self-help groups for all types of women substance users regardless of age, ethnic origins, sexual preference or social class. While the issue of women and substance abuse has already been identified in Afro-Caribbean and Asian cultures (Peckham Black Women's Group and the Alcohol Counselling Service, 1985), the possibility of setting up separate self-help groups for black women and white women is being explored.

The value of this type of work is that women substance abusers, viewed traditionally as a stigmatised, polluted social group, are able within a women-oriented environment to look at the ambiguities, confusion, ambivalence and complexities that underscore their overall human experience and their specific dependence on substances. The sense of isolation experienced previously in private breaks down as women learn to share a renewed sense of vitality and vigour with other women similar to themselves.

On the one hand, by consciously rejecting the victim role, these women gain a new sense of solidarity and strength as women evidence powers uniquely their own. They activate women's praxis. On the other hand, by explicitly accepting the fact that their particular type of experience is grounded in their oppression as women in society, they generate a collective awareness that *all* women need more public and private space to explore what pleases them and to empower themselves as women.

More specifically these women-oriented self-help groups help to create environments in which crucial links between the notions of the private and the public, women and dependency, pollution and femininity and pleasure and danger can be exposed. While the value of these groups must be underscored, there still needs to be more political work, linking these groups with other women's groups. Here it could be argued that the notion of reproduction would be a creative point of linkage, enabling distinct groups of women to organise themselves around a shared basis for the increased development of women's praxis.

Developing feminist strategies: the need for a creative response

What will now be offered is admittedly an exploratory and speculative discussion of the development of feminist strategies in our field of study. Given what has been previously discussed, it may be hoped that we share a profound sense that the women and substance use issue will benefit from an injection of feminist politics, necessitating a clear women-oriented approach. Let us establish the groundwork for this type of politics and see how a feminist analysis has the potential to effect a creative response for women substance users who are viewed in varying degrees as polluted, deviant, outcast women or non-women. With this as our starting point, we continue to lay the foundation for our understanding of women's praxis *vis-à-vis* substance use.

The contention is that specific strategies are needed for the increased emergence of the women and substance use issue specifically within the women's health movement. We will consider a series of key strategies: developing social agency, politicising pollution, seizing the means of reproduction, resisting the transfer of power from the collective to the family, identifying the paradox of social reality, generating a collective consciousness of dependence, deprivatising pain and publicising pleasure, and recognising empowerment as a tool of change. By considering these eight strategies, the discussion explores further the social implications of this issue and attempts to make valuable links with mainstream feminist thought.

Developing social agency

Withstanding powerful dynamics encountered in the field, women substance users should be acutely aware that 'it is not enough to move women away from danger and oppression; it is necessary to move toward something: toward pleasure, agency, self-definition' (Vance, 1984, p. 24). 'Moving towards something' for women substance users is a unique feminist process, already proved successful in the women and health field (Ernst and Maguire, 1987), whereby women develop separate, strong identities within a collective framework. For women substance users this strategy should be a fundamental part of their self-help and feminist practice. Indeed there is a need for a collective context in which women are able to reaffirm their identity as women and to reject wholeheartedly the labels 'junkie', 'food addict', 'alcoholic' or 'tranx addict'.

In developing social agency, women need to recognise that they are, what Lewin (1985, p. 125) refers to as, 'strategic actors':

> Strategic actors . . . select a course of action in the absence of sufficient data . . . the notion that women act in strategic or rational ways in organising their behaviour serves to express by way of analogy the belief that women's behaviour like that of other humans, is created in constant interaction with biological, social and cultural constraints and that outcomes in any and all of those domains may be interpreted to represent a dynamically adaptive process.

The strategies revealed in the ways women use substances are not individually specific and reveal common patterns of experience. It could be argued that women, as strategic actors, choose to use substances as a way of adjusting or modifying their behaviour in response to their oppressive social situations. In this light, their choice is perceived as creative, if not empowering. In other words, it is perceived as a viable course of action in an unpleasant, if not demeaning situation for them as women. To move from being strategic actors towards social agency implies that women substance users first need to recognise why the object of their choice is a substance or substances rather than some other object.

Politicising pollution

Rosaldo (1974, p. 38) has suggested that 'the ideas of purity and pollution, so often used to circumscribe female activities, may also be used as a basis for assertions of female solidarity, power or value'. In this specific context, Rosaldo was highlighting the fact that polluted women who are feared, angry or hold special or anomalous positions in society 'take on powers uniquely their own'. In other words, these women are able to mobilise their own personal power and/or empower themselves by the very fact that they are seen to be polluted.

While these woman are feared, they also have visible personal power and potential collective power. They have this sort of power precisely because the patriarchal system originally devised to maintain order and to control women by separating out what is 'clean' and 'safe' from what is 'dirty' and 'polluted' (Douglas, 1966) has backfired. Perhaps, more poignantly, the male system has turned on itself. In effect, the social dynamics and beliefs surrounding the notion of pollution provide grounds for solidarity among women. Furthermore, extra-domestic ties with other women (such as women's self-help groups) are an important source of power and value in societies that create a firm division between the public and the private spheres (Rosaldo, 1974).

Seizing the means of reproduction

Keeping an awareness of the division between the public and private in mind, women substance users need to develop a thoughtful approach to the notion of reproduction. For example, with the general, uncritical acceptance of FAS (foetal alcohol syndrome) in the field, 'seizing the means of reproduction' has been far from the reach of women substance users. Given that substance use is viewed as damaging to biological and ideological reproduction, women need to clarify the point that this damage is really *social* damage. In other words, substance use is seen to threaten the actual reproduction of labour power as well as the reproduction of relations of production: put simply, substance-using women should not be mothers. If they are, they remain 'unfit mothers' and 'polluted women', capable of 'infecting' their children (born or unborn) with the 'disease' of addiction. In this view, women substance users are unable to educate their children properly in the home (that is, to 'socialise' them). They are unable to prepare them for their future lives as 'productive members of society'. In essence, their children, as social outcasts, are unable to conform to social expectations of what it means to be a principled individual. On some levels, their upbringing is seen as morally reprehensible and tainted with the evil of being born of diseased mothers.

Resisting the transfer of power from the collective to the family

Women's well-being, women's health and women's illness are grounded in their role as dependent care givers. While most of welfare/personal production and reproduction takes place in the home (Rose, 1981, p. 497), it is women who perform this work, at great cost to themselves both physically and mentally. Furthermore poor women and minority women have laboured under a double burden: their bodies have been considered sick and their persons have been considered objects for others use (Hurst and Zambrana, 1980, p. 113). In this context women turn to substances as cushions of support or 'welfare enablers', helping them to perform their work or at least to control and manage their ambivalent feelings about this 'female' work.

Women substance users need to resist the current attempt by 'experts' to transfer the addiction emphasis from society or the collective to the family. In other words the emphasis on the dysfunctional family needs to be challenged in order to gain feminist ground. The dysfunctional family analysis of the addiction problem is dangerous to women because the possibility of making vital links between the public and the private spheres of social life is curtailed. It is only through an awareness of these links that women's praxis on substance use will emerge.

Identifying the paradox of social reality

All women, whether they are substance users or not, are caught up in a paradoxical social reality. On the one hand, women's actual experience of the sexual division of labour remains socially invisible; on the other, what is supposed to be women's normal experience of this division is very visible. For example, while women inhabit a gendered system of domination, they experience a 'fictitious femininity' which is constructed as 'the alleged social norm' and based on the assumption that the sexes have equal status (Enders-Dragaesser, 1988). Women are taught to deny their feelings when these feelings are seen to conflict with what they are supposed to feel. Substance use is one very important way for women to escape from this paradox; it could even be argued that substance use may be perceived as the only means of escape for some women.

We thus see substance use as 'visibly' a vehicle for individual change. However the 'invisible' reality is social transformation: altering the social roles, institutions and systems oppressive to women. As we know already, women substance users are blamed for the negative effects of their substance use; they are stigmatised, told they have an individual problem, victimised by the medical profession, made the targets of various powerful economic interest groups and depoliticised consistently as a potentially powerful group of women. Like all women, women substance users are on the periphery of social power. Additionally, in their quest for social change, they as women have no pre-existing social institutions that they can rely on for social cohesion and collective defence (Lees, 1986, p. 95). By identifying the substance use as an escape from the paradox of their lives, women begin to generate links with other women who experience the paradox of being a woman in society.

Generating a collective consciousness of dependence

In this context women substance users need to develop a collective consciousness of women's dependence experience and to close the gap of social understanding between their normal selves and their addicted selves. Women need to expose collectively both the 'acceptable' and 'unacceptable' faces of dependency and to achieve 'the Courage to See' (Daly, 1988) (that is, the strength to uncover social myths and stereotypes). In other words, women substance users need to become disillusioned, to offer a critical view of who they really are and who they are supposed to be. Their substance use needs to become visible as it is in reality not as it appears through male eyes. Substance use is an integral part of their lives and a piece of all women's dependence experience. In this light, these women have the potential to be capturers of social change, to awaken an awareness of the peripheries and to build potential liberation zones in which women 'recognise themselves, organise themselves, find their common needs and aspirations and find their methods of defense' (Masini, 1981, p. 99).

Given that an understanding of the dual meanings of dependency cannot be isolated from the systems of sex–gender, class and race, women substance users as capturers of social change should emphasise the subtle implications of these meanings. Dependency is a very complex issue, linked with women's being simultaneously depended upon by others. As we already know, giving care and helping others is a fundamental part of a woman's being a dependant. In this light, women substance users need to build 'women spaces' (liberation zones) highlighting the various shades of meanings of dependency on both a public/social and a private/individual level. Organising themselves women substance users will awaken an awareness of their marginality by offering full accounts of their workaday experiences. In a very real sense, the experiences of women substance users are central to the lives of all women.

Deprivatising pain and publicising pleasure

Another challenge for women substance users is to see the potential for effective social action in deprivatising their pain. There exists a real need to make public women's experience of patriarchal pain. Women's substance abuse as a private pleasure is born out of this patriarchal pain encountered by many women. This social, shared pain refers to any of a number of anguishing burdens women carry both publicly and privately in a gendered system of domination. Patriarchal pain is the direct result of the countless contradictions inherent in women's social position.

Pleasure needs to be made public rather than remain hidden below the surface of any woman's inner self. Women use substances because they enjoy it as a pleasurable feeling. Substance use may be a diversion if not an avoidance of patriarchal pain as women struggle to comprehend masculinist reality and their female selves.

There is a need for broader conceptions of substance use which move into the terrain of structure and which uncover ideologies and practices which single out women substance users. Because women have been consistently denied pleasure we need a vision of women as grounded in pleasure. Acknowledging the differences of race, class, culture, age, sexual orientation and ableness amongst women, there is a need to look at the ways in which women can struggle together to replace substance use, a form of pleasurable routine, with *real* feminist affirming practices. As stated in a previous context, while the concept of pleasure for both men and women tends to be linked with sexual achievement and pursuits, pleasure can also be extended to include the notion of empowerment.

Recognising empowerment as a tool of change

Patriarchal power structures tend to confirm masculinist reality, to define who should be at the centre and the peripheries of power and to deny women access to their real women-selves. Women are acutely aware of these debilitating aspects of power. Furthermore, as more women understand the contradictions they confront as women *vis-à-vis* their lack of access to power, they discover the importance of empowerment – particularly the empowerment of women. In discussing this issue, Moglen (1983) identifies the energy behind women's need for empowerment:

> It is this growing recognition of the importance of the special qualities of women's experience that has yielded new significance for 'dailiness' and separation: the wholehearted acceptance by women of their 'proper sphere' as far removed as possible from male hierarchal and authoritarian structures. In this way old wounds are healed and weary spirits strengthened in retreat. (p. 132)

Yet, in a further context, she says:

> Unless we can affirm ourselves and encounter others as 'subjects' . . . in all areas of our lives – we will continue to be subject to all the institutionalized forms of authority which disempower those who are most vulnerable. When they choose to remain outside of that terrain defined as 'male', women choose as well to operate within the boundaries of their own oppression. (p. 132)

Moglen is suggesting that, while women need to celebrate their experiences as women separately from men, real change is found at the boundaries 'in engagement with the centre'. Women need to collect their strength, while at the same time being aware that their strength emerges from within their peripheral status, based on their own social vulnerability.

In this context women substance users must recognise that they are in a position to challenge hierarchal structures of power such as class, gender and race as well as the hierarchy of drugs. While their consciousness of their own vulnerability (their disempowerment) is empowering, they must move towards engagement with the dominant culture in a transformation process. By exposing the structural aspects of their dependency, of both the addiction and the subordinate kind, they offer a captivating position, demystifying the women and substance use issue. While struggling to combat the view that their addiction is an individual problem, they actually make visible the notion that addiction is a social problem as well as a feminist issue.

In conclusion, a basic contention of this chapter has been that developing a feminist perspective on and response to substance use needs thoughtful consideration. Based on a critical analysis of the area of women and substance use, the discussions have illustrated how a review of the varying definitions of substance use as well as the strategies for political action may be a valuable aid to understanding. If women and substance abuse is to be seen as a feminist issue, an awareness of the key political concerns and strategies should be generated in the field. Without this awareness there is a danger that the field of substance abuse will remain politically sterile and insensitive to the needs of women sufferers.

This chapter has been about generating hope. Women substance users, researchers and clinicians – all need to work towards this goal. While hope is based on the belief that 'feminising our worlds' (French, 1984) is a real possibility, it is our skill to make connections, to see our world and to be-witch ourselves. Perhaps more importantly:

> Hope is women's most powerful revolutionary tool; it is what we give each other every time we share our lives, our work and our love. It pulls us forward out of self-hatred, self-blame and the fatalism which keeps us prisoners in separate cells. (Peggy Korneger, quoted in Kramarae and Treichler, 1985, p. 196)

Women substance users need this hope which allows them to see their women-selves as they recognise their close involvement in the sphere of healing. Female energy must be tapped to the full so that hope will become a lived reality rather than a shared vision.

8

Where do we go from here?

> You looked for a flower
> and found a fruit.
> You looked for a well
> and found an ocean.
> You looked for a woman
> and found a soul –
> you are disappointed.

(Edith Sodergran, 'The Day Cools', *Love and Solitude: Selected Poems 1916–1923*, translated by Stina Katchadourian (San Francisco: Fjord Press, 1981))

Introduction

The main aim of this concluding chapter is to weave together some of the key themes developed in the text. The view that there is a need to establish feminist notions in the substance use field in order to be sensitive to the needs of women substance users has been put forward consistently. The substance misuse field needs to be extended beyond its present outdated, boundaries which are insensitive to women. Women substance users need to be removed from being viewed in a negative light. It is hoped that the reader is now aware that this work has made a real attempt to extend boundaries in the field and to initiate a transformation process. This process is concerned with the politicisation of women's substance use or, more precisely, facilitating the development of women and substance use as a feminist issue.

To be alive to feminism in this field is recognise that a women-centred approach is urgently required. Along with this recognition comes an earnest commitment to the concept of 'reflexivity'. In discussing this concept, specifically 'disciplinary reflexivity', Wilkinson (1988, p. 499) notes that 'disciplinary self-awareness is a key factor in the future development of feminist scholarship'. She outlines those strategies capable of challenging dominant paradigms and beneficial to the advancement of feminism. The previous chapter has already explored and outlined in some detail strategies beneficial to the advancement of feminist knowledge and practice in the substance misuse field. The discussion of these strategies implied that a large injection of disciplinary reflexivity is demanded if change for women is to occur. Finally it becomes clearer that defining women substance users' problems and defining women substance users as a problem takes place in a field in which men more than women are the primary definers. Disciplinary reflexivity attempts to challenge this gender imbalance.

Throughout the discussions in this text there has been an engagement in a serious application of this concept of reflexivity. Through the reflective use of 'gender-illuminating notions', discussions have outlined how the women and substance use issue has been defined, the subtle issues which emerge in this defining process and why this issue has been and is defined as a social problem. Our conclusion has consistently been that the issue should become 'visible' as a feminist issue which moves beyond masculinist truths and sees the experience, situations and social positioning of women substance users as a heterogeneous social group. With this visibility the notion that a feminist perspective offers insights into a unique 'way of being in the world' (Stanley, 1990) is further confirmed and understood. Let us now turn our attention to key themes which have been developed in the text.

The quest for pleasure

The quest for pleasure has been linked to women's use of substances. As a deep sense of personal and social satisfaction, based on emotional and physical well-being, pleasure tends to be in small supply in the lives of women substance users, if not of many women. In this wider context Jackson (1984) contends that, given both the social and individual constraints placed upon women, their sexuality and their bodies within a patriarchal society, real pleasure for women is impossible to attain.

Whether or not they use substances, all women need pleasure in their lives. Here the point put forward is that women need to take delight, as men do, in investigating what pleases them and to act in a self-directed and self-centred way. As Webster (1984, p. 393) aptly states, 'the pursuit of pleasure for women makes them feel selfish, unfeminine, not nice'. Likewise women are often afraid to insist on pleasure as a right for themselves. Yet when women take pleasure for themselves, they shift towards a moral stance that affirms the pursuit of pleasure as a more positive value than the pursuit of power. In this context, French (1984) says:

> Patriarchy cannot continue, it cannot survive, if people turn away from power and move toward pleasure. And of all elements on earth, pleasure is the one that is least able to be coerced. People with power can compel behavior, by physical force or threats of punishment of other kinds . . . Authorities can force people to do, to write, to paint, to work a machine. But they cannot force people to feel pleasure . . . They cannot coerce the experience. (pp. 576–7)

Viewed traditionally as self-destructive, a woman's use of substances may also be viewed as an assertive choice and a move towards pleasure. If this is so, she becomes an active consumer and challenges the myths and stereotypes of her as a destructive or out-of-control individual as well as a passive consumer. This active consumption was characterised by women's use of tobacco. Whether or not smoking may be perceived as threatening, active consumption of substances by women tends to be socially threatening. Active consumption challenges social stereotypes of female users. More importantly this process is at the same time a turning away from traditional forms of power and a move towards pleasure. For women, any substance use which actively goes beyond the ideas and practices of women as the controlled and men as the controller spurns traditional forms of power. Women substance users who actively choose pleasure may be saying 'no' to being coerced into a position where pleasure is denied to them.

In this context, let us recall ideas already set out in Chapter 1. By focusing on pleasure, I am looking objectively at whether or not the use of substances contributes to women's sense of well-being. I am *not* advocating substance use. I believe that some if not many women substance users find substance use a form of taking something for themselves. This 'something' not only allows them to feel good, if only in the very short term but also enables them to exert autonomy and, thus, to feel a certain amount of independence from the everyday experience of their own dependence as women. On the other hand, for some women substance users, it is difficult for them to experience autonomy because they validate themselves through relationships with men. As a result they experience low self-esteem, which impedes a sense of their own autonomy (Weiner, Wallen and Zanokowski, 1990).

Nevertheless pleasure for these women is viewed generally as 'more permissible' when it is experienced in relationship to 'dependency of the subordinate thing kind', the 'acceptable face of dependency' rather than in relationship to 'dependency of the addiction kind'. The pleasurable aspects of the latter dependency are often overlooked in the field with the exception of personal accounts of recovery (Harpwood, 1982).

Autonomy and empowerment

While being mindful of the effects of these feminist ideas on the substance use field, let us look at the way the notion of pleasure is linked with autonomy and empowerment.

As more women explore the issue of pleasure it is generally agreed that 'feminism must increase women's pleasure and joy, not just decrease our misery' (Vance, 1984, p. 24). In these explorations, striving for pleasure or a 'quest for pure lust' can be a signal for increasing liberation. For example, the entry for pleasure in the *Feminist Dictionary* says:

> The notion of women taking pleasure is a novel one, in contrast to giving and receiving pleasure. Taking pleasure implies some autonomous activity. (*Diary of a Conference*, quoted in Kramarae and Treichler, 1985, p. 341)

In this context 'taking' appears as a moving towards something (that is, pleasure): a seizure of delight. While implying autonomy, this form of taking suggests at the same time a knowledge of what is pleasurable: one is only able to take something if one knows what that something is and if that something is there to take. But, given that pleasure tends to be a more readily available commodity for men than for women, it may be hard for women to pursue pleasure or to recognise what pleases them, regardless of whether or not pleasure is seen to be in short supply.

While any woman's use of substances can be seen as a move towards pleasure, it is also a step towards breaking down the idea that women substance users are helpless victims. Yet we must be mindful that a woman substance user's experience of pleasure is also mediated by her specific material circumstances (social class, age, race, and so on) as well as her physical and emotional well-being. On the one hand, taking pleasure for a single, white, middle-class western woman may be snorting cocaine at an exclusive penthouse party in the city. On the other hand, a mother from the Yemen may resort to smoking qat as an acceptable way of coping with her workaday village life, riddled with poverty and disease. Whether or not we agree that taking pleasure is concerned with autonomy for women, we should remember that what is 'out there to take' as pleasure, in the form of substances or otherwise varies amongst women.

Women's pleasure seeking must always be balanced against the move towards decreasing pain and degradation for all women. If this balance is not achieved a hierarchy of pleasure, dividing women amongst themselves, will be the end result. Therefore women seeking pleasure must be vigilant of their own needs and the needs of other women. They must consciously move away from what French (1985, p. 577) calls the 'veneration of power', the sense that hierarchy is the only possible way of structuring power in society. Women's access to pleasure varies according to socially constructed hierarchies, ordering the material bases of power. Therefore women must resist replacing these hierarchies with another hierarchy: that of pleasure. The quest for pleasure must be a matter of abolishing hierarchies all together.

Within a feminist context empowerment acts as a safeguard in ensuring that the balance between seeking pleasure and decreasing patriarchal pain is maintained. As a tool of change and a part of women's praxis, empowerment is most definitely a tool of change. It is to do with questioning the continued valuing of hierarchies. As we saw in an earlier context, pleasure for women includes empowerment, activating the feminist process of redefining, experiencing and realising women's own power *vis-à-vis* men.

In the substance use field, empowerment is not only how women in a subordinate social position seek pleasure, it is also breaking down the hierarchy of drugs which involves the ordering of substances from 'good' to 'bad' and less socially polluting to more socially polluting. Seeing, naming and redefining women's substance use means placing a new light on the problems these women may experience in the private sphere. As a result these somewhat intractable problems become more visible in the public domain. In this context empowerment appears as a collective as well as an individual process.

The link between sex and drugs

While the concept of pleasure implies empowerment and autonomy, it is also associated with sexual achievement and conquest for both men and women. This is probably because, of all the pleasures we experience, it could be argued that sex is the most intense, the most profound or the most powerful. It is interesting how, in the substance use field, the pleasure of taking drugs, particularly opiates, has been linked with the pleasure of sex. Exploring this issue, Tom Field (1985, p. 42) says: 'Heroin is nice. Ignoring the consequences and the problems associated with it, the effect of the drug is pleasurable. It is not pleasurable for a certain type of person; it is as generally pleasurable as, say, sex.'

However there exists a substantial amount of mythology around taking heroin as being similar to the 'ultimate orgasm' Stewart (1987, p. 13) notes that, while people have described taking heroin as totally 'euphoric, ecstatic, the best and nicest thing that has ever happened to them', their first experience most probably falls short off this mark. In this context it is suggested that a clearer understanding of substance misuse demands that a break in the link between sex and drugs is made. This link needs to be broken because, for women, the pleasure of sex tends to refer to the pleasure of the male sex or to women's existence as pleasing men and not themselves. In this way, mixing the pleasure of drugs with the pleasure of sex has the potential to be a further denial of women's identity, their existence, and their being as separate from men. Redefining pleasure in a feminist light means that women gain autonomy *vis-à-vis* men. Specifically women substance users need to be seen to exist separately from male substance users: they need to be seen to exist in their own right and for their own physical and psychic integrity.

For example, as a polluted woman with a spoiled identity, the woman heroin user is low on the hierarchy of women generally and women substance users in particular. Being viewed as 'deviant' and 'a whore', she is engaged in using a drug which is seen as low (that is, bad, evil) on the hierarchy of drugs. Perhaps it could be argued that for women, the lower the drug on the hierarchy, the closer the connection exists between them and the 'whore image of women': the more evil the drug appears, the more they are viewed as sexually debased women. Nevertheless, whether women's engagement with drugs is seen to be socially acceptable and 'good' (as with coffee, tea or tranquillisers) or socially unacceptable and 'bad' (heroin, cocaine and so on), any woman's substance use may be seen as a piece of her need for what Daly (1984, p. 80) refers to as 'Physical Ultimacy'. This physical ultimacy is substantially different from physical intimacy or sex.

Physical ultimacy or physical intimacy?

Physical ultimacy demands that women stretch their physical, imaginative, psychic powers beyond the limitations that have been imposed upon them by patriarchal practices. Through physical ultimacy, a woman learns to master herself, rather than be mastered by someone else (a man, men, male superiors, male partners and so on). Physical ultimacy is to do with developing relationships with oneself and others that are 'far-reaching', connecting women with their 'original intuition, the intuition of integrity' (Daly, 1984, p. 81).

In the light of the above, using substances assertively as a way of mastering oneself can be an extremely precarious journey, given the damaging social, psychological and physical consequences of substance use. Women need to replace what is perceived as pleasurable routines (substance use) with life-giving rather than life-threatening practices. What is needed is for women substance users to accept their quest for pleasure, while recognising that substance use can be perceived objectively as one of a limited number of ways for some women to achieve pleasure. They must also be aware that the framework within which they experience this need for pleasure is inexorably linked with their need for empowerment, well-being, creativity, integrity and, ultimately, freedom. Real pleasure and freedom go hand in hand.

Put simply, the quest for women's freedom (liberation) is connected with capturing or perhaps recapturing women's pleasure. In turn this means excavating deep levels of sensuous experiences for women as women. These psychic excavations are focused on claiming women's passion and women's energy as enriching and desirous rather than as destructive and dangerous. Yet the notion of women as the seductive siren and source of evil in the Western Judaeo-Christian culture exists as a powerful image (Prusak, 1974). The power and energy of, as well as the need for, women's pleasure remains subverted, if not denied. However, as more women recognise this energy both on a collective and an individual level, they challenge the subversion and indeed the fear of women's pleasure. These women refuse the 'way of psychic death': an enslavement to men's lust for them. They challenge the way of 'the feminine' in favour of a life filled with pleasure for themselves as women. Asserting women's right to pursue pleasure for themselves, Egerton (1984, p. 202) says:

> Our needs, desires and preferences have all been constructed under male supremacy and our subjective responses to our powerlessness and subordination cannot be prioritised if they further enslave us.

In this way, pursuing pleasure is a full-scale rejection of what it means to be a 'real' woman (that is, a male-oriented and not a woman-oriented woman) in today's society. The feminist quest for pleasure is to do with a woman 'being her own woman' and viewing her sexuality as a bodily and social energy to unite with others (Ferguson, 1989, p. 73).

Decreasing pain

Previous discussions in this text have highlighted the way substance use can be linked with women's experience of what has been referred to as patriarchal pain: the distressing ordeals women experience both publicly and privately in the gendered system of domination. Whether she is a substance user or not, any woman will experience this pain, consciously or unconsciously. By the very fact that she is a woman, this pain is unavoidable for her. In a discussion of female pain, Rich (1976) uses the work of the philosopher–mystic, Simone Weil, who distinguishes between suffering characterised by pain and suffering characterised by affliction, the condition of the oppressed. The former can lead to growth and enlightenment, while the latter is purposeless. Rich says:

> where it is unavoidable, pain can be transformed into something usable, something which takes us beyond the limits of the experience itself into a further grasp of the essentials of life and the possibilities within us. However, over and over she [Weil] equates pure affliction with powerlessness, with waiting, disconnectedness, inertia, the fragmented time of one who is at others' disposal. This insight illuminates much of the female condition. (p. 151–2)

While Rich intended that these ideas be related to the process of giving birth, they can be used in developing our ideas on women and substance use. For example, one can see how a woman substance user is caught up in this process. On the one hand, while her substance use becomes visible in a stressful, painful environment, she may transform this experience of dependency through empowerment; on the other, as a person seen to be 'caring' and engaged in 'labours of love', she is at others' (her childrens' and her husband's) disposal. The irony is that women are not described as labouring when 'we create the essential conditions for the work of men; we are supposed to be acting out of love, instinct, or devotion to some higher cause than self' (Rich, 1979, p. 205).

In this context to be seen to survive, a woman needs to be other-directed rather than self-directed, yet substance use may be perceived as one way for her to be self-directed. For some women it may be the first step towards pleasure, agency or self-definition. For women, to be aware of their deepest desires, to ask for what they want and to get what they want is a taboo that needs to be broken, but to break that taboo is a difficult process. As has been discussed, rather than break that taboo totally, some women use substances as a short-cut to pleasure. They circumvent part of the taboo-breaking route. In other words, because through substance use there may be less of a need for them to ask others directly for what they want, they just do it themselves and take the consequences. It is only when they discover that this self-directed activity may compromise their dependence of the 'subordinate thing kind' that they know they have problems. Their quest for self-direction and independence may turn on themselves.

Thus far women's use of substances has been linked to their need for pleasure. Involving autonomy and empowerment, pleasure was also viewed as an expression of women's need for 'Physical Ultimacy'. This is an 'Elemental' or very deep desire for making real relations with others as well as oneself that are 'far-reaching' powerfully 'intimate' and capable of 'replenishing our innermost Sources' (Daly, 1984, p. 80). Additionally, it was suggested that we need to move towards breaking the link between sex and drugs for women. The implication is that for feminists the notion of 'Physical Ultimacy' could inform the idea and practice of physical intimacy on both a political and an ontological level. With special reference to substance use, connections between Physical Ultimacy and recent feminist discussions concerning the need to re-claim women's bodies and women's sexuality as women should be made. Making these connections allows the reader to delve more deeply into an understanding of the women and substance use issue.

Coming to terms with one's body

In Chapter 6 we saw how women are caught up in a system of bodily subjection and that a woman's relationship to food and her obsession with her body tends to dominate many aspects of her life. The suggestion was that women's bodies are subjected to a politicisation of the body and in turn a politicisation of the soul. For many women their bodies make them feel outsiders in a society in which the simultaneous glorification and degradation of the female form has become a way of life for the insiders in a patriarchal society: men. That 'real' women are only able to assert their bodies as they should be from the point of view of the male gaze rather than as they are with regard to the 'original woman' and their Female Selves should be challenged.

Highlighting this disjunction between the male and the female gaze, Chapkis (1986, p. 5) suggests that any woman's transformation from 'female to feminine' is hard work as well as a mockery. In her view all women need to use the disguise of femininity because their real female selves are unacceptable:

> We are like foreigners attempting to assimilate into a hostile culture, our bodies continually threatening to betray our difference. Each of us who seeks the rights of citizenship through acceptable femininity shares a secret with all who attempt to pass: my undisguised self is unacceptable, I am not what I seem. To successfully pass is to be momentarily wrapped in the protective cover of conformity. To fail is to experience the vulnerability of the outsider. (p. 5)

While the politics of appearance may tell women that their bodies are not quite right for themselves, the politics of substance use tell women that their feelings are not right for themselves. So, to attempt to make the feelings 'right' or perhaps more accurately, to cushion oneself against the 'right' feelings, one comforts one's body with a substance. The body, therefore, is merely a sort of barrier between a woman and the substance that must be conquered rather than 'oneself as not quite right'.

In a real sense, substance use for women may be a way of coming to terms with their own feelings as well as their bodies. An important aspect of substance use is the immediate sense of well-being and/or the feeling that one's problems will be lessened or even solved. Tam Stewart (1987, p. 15) describes her experience of a 'heroin high' and how it allowed her to feel that she could 'take on the world':

> Somewhere deep down in your centre there's a glow, a throb, a tingle. A golden thread runs up your spine and out through the top of your head. A happy smack puppet, warm, comfortable, your body dangles around this taut, buzzing cord. You are stoned. (p. 15)

The author is not advocating that all women should experience this 'heroin high' in order to liberate themselves from the experience of being outsiders in a hostile, male, drug-using culture. Rather the suggestion is that there is a need to recognise that in many aspects of their lives women can be seen to be acting out the need for substance, for validation and for female space. Through substance use, women temporarily lift the weight of a hostile world which separates them from their real female selves.

'Addicting forces' and women

In discussing 'addicting forces' for women in society, O'Sullivan (1987, p. 318) says that addiction often emerges from the 'particular circumstances we are in – many of which are viewed as "normal" and "natural" for women'. While motherhood is viewed as the most natural way of being a woman in society, it is embedded in an ideology which separates sense from emotion and body from mind (Rich, 1976). The implication here is that women's bodies are resources to be used by men to reproduce their (men's) world rather than as they should be: 'sources for women' (Allen, 1986). Women who use substances are seen to abuse their bodies and, more importantly, to damage this important male resource. Pregnant women using substances are made to feel more guilty, shameful and stigmatised than their non-pregnant, substance-using counterparts.

As we saw in Chapter 2, while medical opinion on the use of substances during pregnancy tends to be divided, the consensus appears to be that most, if not all, substance use causes foetal harm. This consensus is set squarely within the institution of medicine which has consistently pathologised pregnancy for women and sees women as a male resource. In this context, Corea (1985) identifies women as being 'mother machines' for men and she notes that reproductive technologies are an increasingly pervasive aspect of women's lives. The point here is that, regardless of whether or not women lose control or appear to lose control of themselves or their bodies through their substance use, women have already lost control of their bodies through the full-scale denial of women's reproductive rights (Arditti, Duelli-Klein and Minden, 1984) and the technological manipulation of women's reproduction (Corea *et al.*, 1985).

Pat Spallone (1989, p. 79) argues that, within the domain of medicine, 'experts' remove the experience of pregnancy and child-birth from women and 'take it out-of-women's-control'. That 80 per cent of pregnant women take prescribed drugs and 35 per cent of pregnant women take a psychoactive drug (Kerns, 1986) indicates a close link between substance use and pregnancy. It may also be a subtle indication of the medical profession's attempt to control women's reproductive experience. On the one hand, women are criticised if they self-prescribe drugs during pregnancy; on the other, they are encouraged to take prescribed drugs offered by their doctor to 'control' this 'condition'. Given that some pregnant woman will often develop psychotic or affective symptoms severe enough to threaten the life of themselves and their foetus, prescribed psychoactive drug use can be seen as a major way of alleviating psychological distress and anxiety, if not a way of forestalling the advance of mental illness (Kerns, 1986). Is it surprising, therefore, that aggressive treatment strategies, such as abortion or sterilisation, have been suggested (Loudon, 1987) as acceptable 'therapeutic' options for these women?

In a real sense, women substance users are seen to be incapable of reproducing fine offsprings. Most women are caught up with 'the primal wish' to have a perfect or at least a non-disabled child (Degener, 1990). Substance-abusing women are excluded from the select pool of 'normal' women who offer genetically and socially 'pure' descendants to society. That this message is visibly eugenic and, additionally, that it pervades most if not all the literature on women, reproduction and substance use is worthy of considerable attention. Although it may not be 'feminine' to express a strong opinion (Brownmiller, 1984, p. 88), women substance users need to be authoritative and to speak from their own experiences as doubly oppressed women. Viewed as reproductively inferior, they need not only to expose how they have been scapegoated as deviant women but also to challenge the eugenic attack on them as subordinate women as compared with 'normal' women.

Given that reproduction is a fundamental human right, women substance users need to counteract the attack on their reproductive freedom. In this context, seizing the means of reproduction, as illustrated in Chapter 7, becomes a key strategy in developing a creative, political response. Asserting the authority of their female selves and their female bodies rather than upholding the authority of the medical profession, these women begin to redefine an understanding of the links between women, reproduction and substance use. Implicitly this process is one of taking damaging practices out of the substance use field as well as recognising the gender-bound construction of knowledge about substance use.

This distinctly feminist process is also one of re-evaluating the world we are wanting to transform as well as the language we use to describe it. As Rich (1979, p. 247) says:

> For many women, the commonest words are having to be sifted through, rejected, laid aside for a long time, or turned to the light for new colors and flashes of meaning: power, love, control, violence, political, personal, private, friendship, community, sexual, work, pain, pleasure, self, integrity . . .

In conclusion, the discussions in this book have attempted to redefine the 'commonest words' with regard to women substance users. They have also served as a conscious way of injecting 'new' (to the field) feminist notions as well as women's praxis into this area. Within a feminist vision, Hite (1987, p. 737) sees that the 'old order' (the male ways of doing things) is crumbling and that everything that seemed permanent and that was taken for granted is now under question. In the light of this vision, this text has been a deliberate attempt to question the fundamental operating principles of the substance use field. To expose and struggle against the invisibility of women's issues in the field is to begin to take women substance users seriously and to be sensitive to their needs. Obviously there is a need for enormous changes in the substance use field in order to nurture a transformative spirit. With this type of transformative spirit in mind, Asphodel (1988, p. 13) aptly says:

> Women as well as men have drunk the poison of patriarchy. We all have to sweat it out, vomit it up, to get rid of it. What does this mean? Simply, that women will have to be recognised and to recognise themselves as normative, powerful members of the human race, not its under half. When this starts, the revolution will really have begun.

As the field begins to cultivate a transformative spirit, clinicians, researchers and substance-using women alike should work towards making the field feminist. The result will be recovery from having drunk the 'poison of patriarchy'. This type of process will mark the beginnings of a shift towards a type of enlightenment, enabling the search for a soul in the field. Searching for and finding a soul will inevitably lead to another discovery: that the desire for true relatedness tends to be hidden in the substance-abuse field. As in society at large, this desire for true relatedness or this wish to love and be loved is often mistaken for dependency and is demeaned in both men and women. True relatedness or authentic loving signifies abundance and not deprivation (McNeely, 1991); it signifies healthy dependence, not unhealthy addiction.

While giving value to relatedness is basic to women, women substance users need to explore their desires for relatedness. On the one hand, they need to look at the fact that they have the potential to relate positively to themselves and to others. On the other hand, they need to assess not only how and why they relate destructively to substances but also where their desire for pleasure can be safely expressed for themselves as women. In this exploration women may find deep disappointment, but they may also find intense satisfaction. Regardless of what unfolds in this exploration, whatever the visible and invisible paths to awareness, women substance users need hope. Whether or not they learn to give up their addictive substances or become less dependent on them, these women need to sense that whomever they approach for help in this field will be sensitive to their needs as women. They need to recognise on what and on whom they can really depend.

Bibliography

Aaro, L., Wood, B., Kanner, L. and Rimpela M. (1984) 'Health Behaviour in School Children: A WHO cross-national study', *Health Promotion*, 1, pp. 17–33.

Action on Alcohol Abuse (1985) personal communication, London.

Action on Smoking and Health (ASH) (1990a) *The Economics of Smoking*, Factsheet No. 3 (London: ASH).

Action on Smoking and Health (1990b) *Women and Tobacco*, Factsheet No. 9 (London: ASH).

Action on Smoking and Health (1990c) *Smoking Statistics*, Factsheet No. 1 (London: ASH).

Ahlstrom, S. (1983) *Women and Alcohol Control Policy: A review of findings and some suggestions for research policy*, Reports from the Social Research Institute of Alcohol Studies, No. 163, Helsinki, Social Research Institute of Alcohol Studies.

Al-Anon Family Groups (1973) *Al-Anon Faces Alcoholism* (New York: Al-Anon Family Group Headquarters, Inc).

Alcoholics Anonymous (1967) *The A.A. Way of Life: a reader by Bill* (London: AA Publishing Company).

Alcohol Concern (1987) *The Drinking Revolution: Building a Campaign for Safer Drinking* (London: Alcohol Concern).

Alcohol Concern (1988) *Women and Drinking* (London: Alcohol Concern).

Alexander, P. (1987) 'Prostitutes are being Scapegoated for Heterosexual AIDS', in F. Delacoste and P. Alexander (eds) *Sex Work: Writings by Women in the Sex Industry* (London: Virago) pp. 248–63.

Alexander, P. (1988) 'A Chronology, of Sorts', in I. Rieder and P. Ruppelt (eds) *AIDS: The Women* (San Francisco: Cleis Press) pp. 169–72.

Allan, C. (1987) 'Seeking Help for Drinking Problems from a Community-based Voluntary Agency. Patterns of Compliance amongst men and women', *British Journal of Addiction*, 82, pp. 1143–7.

Allan, C. and Cooke D. (1986) 'Women, Life Events and Drinking Problems' *British Journal of Psychiatry*, 148, pp. 460–5.

Allen, J. (1986) *Lesbian Philosophy: Explorations* (Palo Alto, California: Institute of Lesbian Studies).

Annis, H. M. and Liban, C. B. (1980) 'Alcoholism in Women: Treatment Modalities and Outcomes', in Oriana Josseau Kalant (ed.) *Alcohol and Drug Problems in Women* (London: Plenum Press) pp. 385–422.

Appel, C. (1990) 'Women, Alcohol and Society', paper presented to the 16th Annual Alcohol Epidemiology Symposium, Budapest, Hungary, 3–8 June 1990.

Arber, S. (1990) Revealing Women's Health: Re-analysing the General Household Survey in H. Roberts (ed.) *Women's Health Courts* (London: Routledge pp. 66–92).

Ardener, E. (1975) 'Belief and the Problem of Women', in Shirley Ardener (ed.) *Perceiving Women* (London: J. M. Dent & Sons Ltd) pp. 1–17.

Arditti, R., Duelli-Klein, R. and Minden, S. (1984) *Test-Tube Women* (London, Pandora Press).

Aristophanes, *Lysistrata.*

Ashton, H. and Golding, J. (1989) 'Tranquillisers: Prevalence, predictors and possible consequences. Data from a large United Kingdom survey', *British Journal of Addiction*, 84, 5, pp. 541–6.

Ashton, H. and Stepney, R. (1982) *Smoking Psychology and Pharmacology* (London: Tavistock).

Asphodel (1988) '1968: Prague Winter, Feminist Spring', in A. Sebestyen (ed.) *'68, '78, '88: From Women's Liberation to Feminism* (Bridport, Dorset: Prism Press) pp. 7–14.

Association of the British Pharmaceutical Industry (1986a) *Careers in Pharmaceuticals* (London: ABPI).

Association of the British Pharmaceutical Industry (1986b) *The UK Pharmaceutical Industry: Facts '86* (London: ABPI).

Association of the British Pharmaceutical Industry (1987) *Annual Report 1986–87* (London: ABPI).

Bardsley, B. (1984) 'The Incurable Illness', in H. Kanter, S. Lefanu, S. Shah and C. Spedding (eds) *Sweeping Statements: Writings from the Women's Liberation Movement 198-83* (London: Women's Press) pp. 205–9.

Barrett, M. and Roberts, H. (1978) 'Doctors and Their Patients: The Social Control of Women in General Practice', in C. Smart and B. Smart (eds) *Women, Sexuality and Social Control* (London: Routledge & Kegan Paul) pp. 41–52.

Bas Hannah, S. (1983) 'whoever i am i'm a fat woman', in L. Schoenfielder and B. Wieser (eds) *Shadow on a Tightrope* (Iowa City: Aunt Lute Books) pp. xxiv-vi.

Beckman, L. (1975) 'Women Alcoholics: A review of social and psychological studies', *Journal of the Study of Alcohol* 36, pp. 797–824.

Beckman, L. (1978) 'The self-esteem of women alcoholics', *Journal of Studies on Alcohol*, 39, 3, pp. 491–8.

Beckman, L. (1980) 'Perceived antecedents and effects of alcohol consumption in women', *Quarterly Journal of the Study of Alcohol*, 41, 5, pp. 518–30.

Beckman, L. (1984) 'Treatment needs of women alcoholics', *Alcoholism Treatment Quarterly*, 1, 2, pp. 101–15.

Beckman, L. and Amaro, H. (1984) 'Patterns of women's use of alcohol treatment agencies', in S. C. Wilsnack and L. Beckman (eds) *Alcohol Problems in Women* (New York: Guilford Press).

Beechey, V. (1986) 'Women's Employment in Contemporary Britain', in V. Beechey and E. Whitelegg (eds) *Women in Britain Today* (Milton Keynes: Open University Press) pp. 77–131.

Bejerot, N. (1980) 'Addiction to Pleasure: A Biological and Social-Psychological Theory of Addiction', in D. J. Lettieri, M. Sayers and H. W. Pearson (eds) *Theories on drug abuse: selected contemporary perspectives* (Rockville, Maryland: NIDA) pp. 246–55.

Bellantuono, C. *et al.* (1980) 'Benzodiazepines: Clinical Pharmacology and Therapeutic Use', *Drugs*, 19, pp. 195–219.

Belle, D. (1984) 'Inequality and Mental Health: Low Income and Minority Women' in L. A. Walker (ed.) *Women and Mental Health Policy* (Beverley Hills: Sage Publications) pp. 135–50.

Berridge, V. (1988) 'The Origins of the English Drug Scene: 1890–1930', *Medical History*, 32, pp. 51–64.

Berridge, V. and Edwards, G. (1981) *Opium and the People* (London: Allen Lane and New York: St. Martin's Press).

Black, D. (1988) 'Temazepam capsules', *Lancet*, 1, 8594, p. 1114.

Blume, S. B. (1990a) 'Chemical Dependency in Women: Important Issues', *American Journal of Drug and Alcohol Abuse*, 16 (3 and 4) pp. 297–307.

Blume, S. B. (1990b) 'Alcohol and Drug Problems in Women: Old Attitudes, New Knowledge', in H. B. Milkman and L. I. Sederer (eds) *Treatment Choices for Alcoholism and Substance Abuse* (Lexington, DC: Heath and Company) pp. 183–200.

Boskind-Lodahl, M. (1976) 'Cinderella's stepsisters: A feminist perspective on anorexia nervosa and bulimia', *SIGNS: Journal of Women in Culture and Society*, 2, pp. 341–56.

Boskind-White, J. (1981) 'Fat: A Feminist Issue', *Focus on Women*, 2, 1, pp. 48–55.

Boston Women's Health Collective (1971) *Our Bodies Ourselves: A Book by and for Women* (New York, Simon & Schuster).

Boston Women's Health Collective (1978) A. Phillips and J. Rakusen (eds) *Our Bodies Ourselves: A Book By and for Women*, British Edn (Harmondsworth: Penguin).

Bovery, S. (1989) *Being Fat is Not a Sin* (London: Women's Press).

Bradshaw, J. (1988) *Healing the Shame that Binds You* (Dearfiled Beach, Florida: Health Communications Inc).

Brazier, C. (1988) 'The Politics of Greed and the Path Beyond', *New Internationalist*, 188, pp. 4–6.

Breeze, E. (1985) *Women and Drinking* (London: HMSO).

Brooks, J. (1953) *The Mighty Leaf: Tobacco Through the Centuries* (London: Alvin Redman Limited).

Brown, C. (1984) *Black and White Britain* (London: Gower).

Brown, G. W. and Harris, T. (1978) *Social Origins of Depression: A study of psychiatric disorders in women* (London: Tavistock).

Brown, L. S. (1987) 'Lesbians, Weight, and Eating: New analyses and Perspectives', in Boston Lesbian Psychologies Collective (ed.) *Lesbian Psychologies: Explorations and Challenges* (Chicago: University of Illinois Press) pp. 294–309.

Brown, V., Manderson, D., O'Callaghan, M. and Thompson, R. (1986) *Our Daily Fix: Drugs in Australia* (Ruschuttes Bay, New South Wales: Pergamon Press).

Brownlee, R. (1981) 'Issues Surrounding the Woman Administrator in Drug Abuse', in A. J. Schecter (ed.) *Drug Dependence and Alcoholism, Volume 1: Biomedical Issues* (New York: Plenum Press) pp. 935–43.

Brownmiller, S. (1984) *Femininity* (London: Paladin, Grafton Books).

Bruegel, I. (1982) 'Women as a Reserve Army of Labour: A Note on Recent British Experience', in E. Whitelegg *et al.* (eds) *The Changing Experience of Women* (Oxford: Basil Blaskwell in association with the Open University).

Bruun, K. (ed.) (1982) *Alcohol, Control Policies in the United Kingdom* (Stockholm: Sociologiska Institutionen).

Bryan, B., Dadzie, S. and Scafe, S. (1985) *The Heart of the Race: Black Women's Lives in Britain* (London: Virago).

Burbank, F. (1972) 'US lung cancer death rates begin to rise proportionately more rapidly for females than for males: A dose-response effect?', *Journal of Chronic Diseases*, 25, pp. 473–9.

Burr, A. (1985) 'The Ideologies of Despair: A Symbolic Interpretation of Punks and Skinheads' Use of Barbiturates, *Social Science and Medicine*, 19, 9, pp. 929–38.

Burtle, V. (ed.) (1979) *Women Who Drink* (Springfield Mass.: Thomas).

Bury, M. and Gabe, J. (1990) 'A Sociological View of Tranquilliser Dependence: Challenges and Responses', in I. Hindmarch, G. Beaumont, S. Brandon and B. E.Leonard (eds) *Benzodiazepines: Current Concepts* (New York: John Wiley) pp. 211–25.

Butler, J. (1987) 'Variations on Sex and Gender: Beauvoir, Wittig and Foucault', in S. Benhabib and D. Cornell (eds) *Feminism as Critique* (Cambridge: Polity Press) pp. 128–42.

Butt, Louise (1989) 'Women and AIDS', *Connexions: The Journal of Drug and Alcohol Issues*, May/June, 9, 3, pp. 27–32.

Camberwell Council on Alcoholism (1980) *Women and Alcohol* (London: Tavistock).

Carby, H. V. (1982) 'Schooling in Babylon', in Centre for Contemporary Cultural Studies *The Empire Strikes Back: Race and Racism in 70s Britain* (London: Hutchinson) pp. 183–211.

Cavanagh, J. and Clairmonte, F. (1985) *Alcoholic Beverages: Dimensions of Corporate Power* (London: Croom Helm).

Central Policy Review Staff (1979) *Alcohol Control Policies in the United Kingdom*, available from Stockholm: Sociologiska Institutionen (see Bruun, K. (ed.) 1982).

Chapkis, W. (1986) *Women and the Politics of Appearance* (London: Women's Press).

Chernin, K. (1981) *Womansize: The Tyranny of Slenderness* (London: Women's Press).

Chernin, K. (1985) *The Hungry Self: Women, Eating and Identity* (London: Virago).

Chesler, P. (1972) *Women and Madness* (New York: Avon Books).

Chein, I., Gerard, D. L., Lee, R. S. and Rosenfeld, E. (1964) *The Road to H: Narcotics, Delinquency and Social Policy* (New York: Basic Books).

Chick, J. (1985) 'Some Requirements of an Alcohol Dependence Syndrome', in N. Heather, I. Robertson and P. Davies (eds) *The Misuse of Alcohol* (London: Croom Helm) pp. 45–58.

Chodorow, N. (1978) *The Reproduction of Mothering* (Berkeley: University of California Press).

CIBA FOUNDATION (1984) *Mechanisms of Alcohol Damage in Utero*, Symposium 105 (London: Pitman).

Clare, A. (1981) 'Psychotropic Drug Use in General Practice', in G. Tognoni, C. Bellantuono and M. Lader (eds) *Epidemiological Impact of Psychotropic Drugs* (Amsterdam: Elsevier/North Holland Biomedical Press) pp. 189–201.

Cohen, J., Alexander, P. and Wofsy, C. (1988) 'Prostitutes and AIDS: Public Policy Issues', *AIDS and Public Policy Journal*, 3, 2, pp. 16–22.

Cohen, S. (1981) *The Substance Abuse Problems* (New York: Haworth Press).

Colton, M. E. (1981) 'A Description and Comparative Analysis of Self-Perceptions and Attitudes of Heroin-Addicted Women', in A. J. Schecter (ed.) *Drug Dependence and Alcoholism Volume 1: Biomedical Issues* (New York: Plenum Press) pp. 927–33.

Committee on the Review of Medicines (1980) Systematic Review of the Benzodiazepines, *British Medical Journal*, 29: 910–2.

Committee on the Safety of Medicines (1988) 'Benzodiazepines, dependence and withdrawal symptoms', *Current Problems*, 21.

Connor, B. and Babcock, M. (1980) 'The Impact of Feminist Psychotherapy on the Treatment of Women Alcoholics', *Focus on Women: Journal of Addictions and Health*, 1, 2, pp. 77–92.

Cooke, D. J. and Allan, C. A. (1984) 'Stressful Life Events and Alcohol Abuse in Women: A General Population Study', *British of Journal of Addiction* 79, 4, pp. 425–30.

Cooperstock, R. and Lennard, H. L. (1986) 'Some Social Meanings of Tranquilliser Use', in J. Gabe and P. Williams (eds) *Tranquillisers: Social, Psychological and Clinical Perspectives* (London: Tavistock) pp. 227–43.

Cooperstock, R. and Parnell, P. (1982) 'Research on psychotropic drug use', *Social Science and Medicines*, 16, pp. 1179–96.

Corea, G. (1985) *The Mother Machine* (London: Women's Press).

Corea, G., Duelli-Klein, R., Hanmer, J., Holmes, H. B., Hoskins, B., Kishwar, M., Raymond, J., Rowland, R. and Steinbacher, R. (1985) *Man-Made Women* (London: Hutchinson).

Corrigan, E. (1980) *Alcoholic Women in Treatment* (New York: Oxford University Press).

Corrigan, E. and Anderson, S. C. (1982) 'Black Alcoholic Women in Treatment', *Focus on Women: Journal of Addiction and Health*, 3, 1, pp. 49–58.

Craig, M., Cappell, H., Busto, U. and Kay, G. (1987) 'Cognitive–Behavioural Treatment for Benzodiazepine Dependence: A comparison of gradual versus abrupt cessation of drug intake', *British Journal of Addiction*, 82, pp. 1317–27.

Crisp, L. (1984) 'Women and Addiction', *The National Times* (Australia) 23–9 November, pp. 16 and 18.

Curlee, J. (1968) 'Women Alcoholics', *Federal Probation*, 32, pp. 16–20.

Curlee, J. (1969) 'Alcoholism and the "empty nest"', *Bulletin of the Menniger Clinic*, 33, pp. 165–71.

Curlee, J. (1970) 'A comparison of male and female patients at an alcoholism treatment centre', *Journal of Psychology*, 74, pp. 239–47.

Curran, V. and Golombok, S. (1985) *Bottling it Up* (London: Faber & Faber).

Cuskey, W. R. (1982) 'Female Addiction: A Review of the Literature', *Focus on Women: Journal of Addiction and Health*, 13, 1, pp. 3–33.

Cuskey, W. R., Berger, L. H., and Densen-Gerber, J. (1977) 'Issues in the treatment of female addiction: a review and critique of the literature', *Contemporary Drug Problems*, 6,3, pp. 307–72.

Cyr, M. G. and Moulton, A. W. (1990) 'Substance Abuse in Women', *Obstetrics and Gynecology Clinics of North America*, 17, 4, pp. 905–25.

Daily Mail (1987) Thursday 13 November, p. 6.

Daly, M. (1984) *Pure Lust: Elemental Feminist Philosophy* (London: Women's Press).

Daly, M. in cahoots with J. Caputi (1988) *Webster's First New Intergalactic WICKEDARY of the English Language* (London: Women's Press).

Dan, M., Rock, M. and Bar-Shani, S. (1987) 'HIV Antibodies in Drug Addicted Prostitutes', *Journal of American Medical Association* 257, 8: 1047.

DAWN (1984) *Women and Heroin* (London: DAWN).

DAWN (1985a) *Women and Alcohol* (London: DAWN).

DAWN (1985b) *Women and Tranquillisers* (London: DAWN).

DAWN (1985c) *Survey of Facilities for Women using Drugs (including alcohol) in London* (London: DAWN).

DAWN (1986) *Women and Stimulants* (London: DAWN).

DAWN (1988a) *HIV and AIDS: Facts for women who use drugs* (London: DAWN).

DAWN (1988a) *Women and Smoking*. London, DAWN.

Day, S. (1988) 'Prostitute Women and AIDS: anthropology', *AIDS*, 2, 6, pp. 421–7.

Day, S. and Ward, H. (1990) 'The Praed Street Project: a cohort of prostitute women in London', in M. Plant (ed.) *Aids, Drugs and Prostitution* (London: Routledge) pp. 61–75.

Degener, T. (1990) 'Female self-determination between feminist claims and "voluntary" eugenics, between "rights" and ethics', *Reproductive and Genetic Engineering*, 3, 2, pp. 87–99.

Delacoste, F. and Alexander, P. (eds) (1987) *Sex Work: Writings by Women in the Sex Industry* (London: Virago).

Delphy, C. (1984) *Close to Home: A Materialist analysis of Women's Oppression* (London: Hutchinson).

Diamond, J. (1987) 'Foreword', in *Annual Report 1986–87* (London: ABPI) p. 3.

Diamond, N. (1985) 'Thin is the Feminist Issue', *Feminist Review*, 19, pp. 45–64.

Dickenson, J. (1983) 'Some Thoughts on Fat', in L. Schoenfielder and Barb Wieser (eds) *Shadow on a Tightrope* (Iowa City: Aunt Lute Book Company) pp. 37–51.

Dixon, A. (1987) 'The Pregnant Addict', *Druglink*, 2, 4, pp. 6–8.

Doll, R. and Hill, A. B. (1950) 'Smoking and Carcinoma of the Lung', *British Medical Journal*, 2, pp. 739–48.

Dorn, N. (1980) 'The Conservatism of the Cannabis Debate', in National Deviancy Conference (ed.) *Permissiveness and Control: The Fate of Sixties Legislation* (London: Macmillan) pp. 44–71.

Dorn, N. and South, N. (1989) 'Drugs and Leisure, Prohibition and Pleasure: From Subculture to Drugalogue', in C. Rojek (ed.) *Leisure for Leisure* (London: Macmillan) pp. 171–90.

Douglas, M. (1966) *Purity and Danger* (London: Routledge & Kegan Paul).

Doyal, L. (1981) *The Political Economy of Health* (London: Pluto Press).

Doyal, L. (1983) 'Women, Health and the Sexual Division of Labour: A Case Study of the Women's Health Movement in Britain', *International Journal of Health Services*, 13, 3, pp. 373–87.

Doyal, L. and Elston, M. (1986) 'Women, Health and Medicine', in V. Beechey and E. Whitelegg (eds) *Women in Britain Today* (Milton Keynes: Open University Press) pp. 173–209.

Duckert, F. (1984) 'Evaluation of Treatment for Female Problem Drinkers', paper presented at the Third International Conference on Treatment and Addictive Behaviours, North Berwick, Scotland, 12–16 August.

Duckert, F. (1988) 'Recruitment to Alcohol Treatment: A comparison between male and female problem drinkers recruited to treatment in two different ways', *British Journal of Addiction*, 83, 3, pp. 285–93.

Duelli-Klein, R. (1983) 'How to do what we want to do: thoughts about feminist methodology', in G. Bowles and R. Duelli-Klein (eds) *Theories of Women's Studies* (London: Routledge & Kegan Paul) pp. 88–104.

DuPont, R. (1990) 'Benzodiazepines and Chemical Dependence: Guidleines for Clinicians', *Substance Abuse*, 11, 4, pp. 232–6.

Dworkin, A. (1987) *Intercourse* (London: Secker & Warburg).

Edwards, G. (1977) 'The alcohol dependence syndrome: usefulness of an idea', in G. Edwards and M. Grant (eds) *Alcoholism: New Knowledge and New Responses* (London: Croom Helm).

Edwards, G. (1978) 'Drugs, and the Questions that can be Asked of Epidemiology', in J. Fishman (ed.) *The Bases of Addiction* (Berlin: Dahlem Konferenzen).

Edwards, G. (1980) 'Alcoholism treatment: between guesswork and certainty', in G. Edwards and M. Grant (eds) *Alcoholism Treatment in Transition* (London: Croom Helm).

Edwards, G. (1982) *The Treatment of Drinking Problems: a Guide for the Helping Professions* (London: Grant McIntyre Medical and Scientific).

Edwards, G. (1984) 'Addiction: A Challenge to Society', *New Society,* 25 October 1984, pp. 133–5.

Edwards, G. and Gross, M. (1976) 'Alcohol dependence: provisional description of a clinical syndrome', *British Medical Journal,* i, pp. 1058–61.

Egerton, J. (1984) 'The Goal of Feminist Politics . . . The Destruction of Male Supremacy or the Pursuit of Pleasure? A Critique of the Sex Issue of Heresies', in H. Kanter, S. Lefanu, S. Shah and C. Spedding (eds) *Sweeping Statements: Writings from the Women's Liberation Movement 1981–83* (London: Women's Press) pp. 198–202.

Ehrenreich, B. and English, D. (1974) *Complaints and Disorders: The Sexual Politics of Sickness* (London: Compendium).

Einstein, S. (1983) 'Self-Help Drug Misuse Intervention: A Schema', *International Journal of the Addictions,* 18, 4, pp. 559–68.

Enders-Dragaesser, U. (1988) 'Women's identity and development within a paradoxical reality', *Women's Studies International Forum,* 11, 6, pp. 583–90.

English Collective of Prostitutes (1987) *Prostitute Women and AIDS: Resisting the Virus of Repression* (London: English Collective of Prostitutes).

Erickson, P. G. and Watson, V. A. (1990) 'Women, Illicit Drugs and Crime', in L. Kozlowski, H. Annis, H. Cappell, F. Glaser, M. Goodstadt, Y. Israel, H. Kalant, E. Seelers and E. Vingilis (eds) *Research Advances in Alcohol and Drug Problems* (New York: Plenum Press) pp. 251–72.

Ernst, S. and Goodison, L. (1981) *In Our Own Hands: A Book of Self-Help Therapy* (London: Women's Press).

Ernst, S. and Maguire, M. (1987) 'Introduction: Living the Question', in S. Ernst and M. Maguire (eds) *Living with the Sphinx* (London: The Women's Press).

Estep, R. (1987) 'The Influence of the Family on the Use of Alcohol and Prescription Depressants by Women', *Journal of Psychoactive Drugs,* 19, 2, pp. 171–9.

Ettorre, E. M. (1984) 'A Study of Alcoholism Treatment Units: Treatment Activities and the Institutional Response', *Alcohol and Alcoholism,* 19, pp. 243–55.

Ettorre, E. M. (1985a) 'A Study of Alcoholism Treatment Units: Links with the Community', *British Journal of Addiction,* 79, pp. 181–9.

Ettorre, E. M. (1985b) 'A Study of Alcoholism Treatment Units: Some Findings on Unit and Staff', *Alcohol and Alcoholism,* 20, pp. 371–8.

Ettorre, E. M. (1985c) 'A Study of Alcoholism Treatment Units: Some Findings on Patients', *Alcohol and Alcoholism,* 20, pp. 361–9.

Ettorre E. M. (1985d) 'Psychotropics, Passivity and the Pharmaceutical Industry', in Anthony Henman, Roger Lewis and Tim Maylon (eds) *The Big Deal: the politics of the illicit drugs business* (London: Pluto Press).

Ettorre, B. (1986a) 'Women and Drunken Sociology: Developing a Feminist Analysis', *Women's Studies International Forum,* 9, 5, pp. 515–20.

Ettorre, E. M. (1986b) 'Self-Help Groups as an Alternative to Benzodiaze-pine Use', in J. Gabe and P. Williams (eds) *Tranquillisers: Social, Psychological and Clinical Perspectives* (London: Tavistock) pp. 180–93.

Ettorre, B. (1989a) 'Women, Substance Abuse and Self-Help', in S. MacGregor (ed.) *Drugs and British Society* (London: Routledge).

Ettorre, B. (1989b) 'Women and Substance Abuse: Towards a Feminist Perspective or How to Make Dust Fly', *Women's Studies International Forum*, 12,6, pp. 593–602.

Farrell, M. and Strang, J. (1988) 'Misuse of temazepam', *British Medical Journal*, 297, 6660, p. 1402.

Ferguson, A. (1989) *Blood at the Root: Motherhood, Sexuality and Male Dominance* (London: Pandora).

Ferrence, R. G. (1980) 'Sex Differences in the Prevalence of Problem Drinking', in O. J. Kalant (ed.) *Alcohol and Drug Problems in Women* (New York and London: Plenum Press) pp. 69–124.

Field, T. (1985) *Escaping the Dragon* (London: Unwin Paperbacks).

Fillmore, K. M. (1984a) 'When Angels Fall: Women's Drinking as Cultural Preoccupation and as Reality', in S. C. Wilsnack and L. Beckman (eds) *Alcohol Problems in Women: Antecedents, Consequences* (New York: The Guilford Press) pp. 7–36.

Fillmore, K. M. (1984b) 'The epidemiology of alcohol abuse among women: A history of science approach', *Bulletin of the Society of Psychologists in Addictive Behaviors*, 3, 3, pp. 130–6.

Fillmore, K. M. (1987) 'Women's drinking across the adult life course as compared with men's', *British Journal of Addiction*, 82, pp. 801–11.

Finch, J. and Groves, D. (1982) 'By women for women: caring for the frail elderly', *Women's Studies International Forum*, 5, p. 5.

Finnegan, D. G. and McNally, E. B. (1987) *Dual Identities: Counselling Chemically dependent Gay Men and Lesbians* (Hazelden: Hazelden Press).

Fortney, D. (1990) 'Drug Use in Pregnancy', *Minnesota Medicine*, 73 (4) pp. 41–3.

Foucault, M. (1977) *Discipline and Punish: The Birth of a Prison* (Harmondsworth: Penguin Books).

French, M. (1984) *Beyond Power: On Women, Men and Morals* (London: Sphere Books).

Fruchter, R. G., Fatt, N., Booth, P. and Leidel, D. (1977) 'The Women's Health Movement: Where are we Now?', in C. Dreifus (ed.) *Seizing our Bodies: The Politics of Women's Health* (New York: Vintage Books) pp. 271–8.

Fursland, A. (1987) 'Eve was Framed: Food and Sex and Women's Shame', in M. Lawrence (ed.) *Fed Up and Hungry: Women, Oppression and Food* (London: Women's Press) pp. 15–26.

Gabe, J. (1990) 'Towards a sociology of tranquilliser prescribing', *British Journal of Addiction*, 85, 1, pp. 41–8.

Gabe, J. and Lipshitz-Phillips, S. (1982) 'Evil Necessity? The meaning of benzodiazepine use for women patients from one general practice', in *Sociology of Health and Illness*, 2, 4, pp. 201–9.

Gabe, J. and Lipshitz-Phillips, S. (1984) 'Tranquillisers as Social Control?', *Sociological Review*, 32, 3, pp. 524–46.

Gabe, J. and Thorogood, N. (1986a) 'Tranquillisers as a Resource', in J. Gabe and P. Williams (eds) *Tranquillisers: Social, Psychological and Clinical Perspectives* (London: Tavistock) pp. 244–69.

Gabe, J. and Thorogood, N. (1986b) 'Prescribed drug use and the management of everyday life: the experiences of black and white working-class women', *Sociological Review*, 34, pp. 737–72.

Gabe, J. and Williams, P. (1986) 'Tranquilliser Use: a historical perspective', in J. Gabe and P. Williams (eds) *Tranquillisers: Social, Psychological and Clinical Perspectives* (London: Tavistock) pp. 3–17.

Gallager, J. (1987) 'Eggs, Embryos and Foetuses: Anxiety and the Law', in M. Stanworth (ed.) *Reproductive Technologies: Gender, Motherhood and Medicine* (Cambridge: Polity Press) pp. 139–50.

Garmarnikow, E., Morgan, D., Purvis, J. and Taylorson, D. (eds) (1983) *The Public and the Private* (London: Heineman).

Gilligan, C. (1982) *In a Different Voice* (Cambridge, Mass.: Harvard University Press).

Glasser, W. (1976) *Positive Addiction* (New York: Harper & Row).

Glatt, M. (1974) *A Guide to Addiction and its Treatment* (Lancaster: Medical and Technical Publishing Company Limited).

Glatt, M. (1975) *Alcoholism – A Social Disease* (London: Teach Yourself Books).

Glendenning, M. and Laing, W. (1987) *The Politics of Health Care* (London: ABPI).

Glover Reed, B. (1987) 'Developing Women-Sensitive Drug Dependence Treatment Services: Why so Difficult?', *Journal of Psychoactive Drugs*, 19, 2, pp. 151–64.

Gofton, L. (1983) 'Real Ale and Real Men', *New Society*, 66, 1096, pp. 271–3.

Golombok, S. (1991) 'The contribution of psychology to understanding long-term tranquilliser use', in J. Gabe (ed.) *Understanding Tranquilliser Use: the role of the social sciences* (London: Tavistock/Routledge) pp. 15–30.

Gomberg, E. (1974) 'Women and Alcoholism', in V. Franks and V. Burtle (eds) *Women in Therapy: New Psychotherapies for a Changing Society* (New York: Brunner/Masel) pp. 169–90.

Gomberg, E. (1976) 'Alcoholism in Women', in B. Kissin and H. Begleiter (eds) *The Biology of Alcoholism, Vol. 4: Social Aspects of Alcoholism* (New York: Plenum Press) pp. 117–66.

Gomberg, E. (1979) 'Drinking patterns of women alcoholics', in V. Burtle (ed.) *Women who Drink* (Springfield Mass.: Thomas).

Gordon, B. (1979) *I'm Dancing as Fast as I Can* (London: Hamish Hamilton).

Gossop, M. (1982) *Living with Drugs*, 1st edn (London: Temple Smith).

Graham, H. (1983) 'Caring: a labour of love', in J. Finch and D. Groves (eds) *A Labour of Love: Women, Work and Caring* (London: Routledge) pp. 13–30.

Graham, H. (1984) *Women, Health and the Family* (Brighton: Wheatsheaf).

Graham, H. (1987) 'Women's Smoking and Family Health'. *Social Science and Medicine*, 25, 1, pp. 47–56.

Graham, H. (1990) 'Behaving well: women's health behaviour in context', in H. Roberts (ed.) *Women's Health Counts* (London: Routledge) pp. 195–219.

Graham, H. (1991) 'The Concept of Caring in Feminist Research: the case of domestic service', *Sociology*, 25,1, pp. 61–78.

Greenblatt, M. and Schuckit, M. A. (1976) *Alcoholism Problems in Women and Children* (New York: Grune and Stratton).

Griffin, S. (1978) *Woman and Nature: The Roaring Inside Her* (London: Women's Press).

Griffin, S. (1981) *Pornography and Silence: Culture's Revenge against Nature* (London: Women's Press).

Gritz, E. R. (1980) 'Problems Related to Use of Tobacco by Women', in O. J. Kalant (ed.) *Alcohol and Drug Problems in Women* (London: Plenum Press) pp. 487–543.

Hall, N. (1980) *The Moon and the Virgin* (London: Women's Press).

Hallstrom, C. (1989) 'Benzodiazepines – The Medical View', in *SCODA Newsletter*, September–October, pp. 12–13.

Hamburger, W. W. (1951) 'Emotional aspects of obesity', in *Medical Clinician of North America*, 35, pp. 483–99.

Hankin, R. (1988) *European Regulations* (London: ABPI).

Hanmer, J. (1985) 'Transforming consciousness: women and the new reproductive technologies', in G. Corea *et al.* (eds) *Man-Made Women* (London: Hutchinson).

Harding, S. and Hintikka, M. B. (eds) (1983) *Discovering Reality: Feminist Perspectives on Epidemiology, Metaphysics, Methodology and Philosophy of Science* (Boston: D. Reidel).

Harpwood, D. (1982) *Tea and Tranquillisers* (London: Virago).

Harrison, P. A. and Belille, C. A. (1987) 'Women in treatment: beyond the stereotype', *Journal of Studies on Alcohol*, 48, pp. 574–8.

Harwin, J. and Otto, S. (1979) 'Women, Alcohol and the Screen', in J. Cook and M. Lewington (eds) *Images of Alcoholism* (London: British Film Institute and Alcohol Education Centre) pp. 37–50.

Hatsukami, D. K. and Owen, P. (1982) 'Social Roles and Treatment Outcome in Women with Alcohol or Drug Abuse Problems', *Focus on Women: Journal of Addiction and Health*, 3, 2, pp. 118–23.

Hawkins, J. (1976) 'Lesbianism and Alcoholism', in M. Greenblatt and M. A. Schuckit, *Alcoholism Problems in Women and Children* (New York: Grune and Stratton) pp. 137–54.

Healy, P. (1980) 'Pan Pacific Conference on Drugs and Alcohol, The Pregnant Pause Campaign: An Explanation and Outline', *Focus on Women: Journal on Addiction and Health*, 1, 3, pp. 204–13.

Heather, N. (1985) 'Introduction', in N. Heather, I. Robertson and P. Davies (eds) *The Misuse of Alcohol* (London: Croom Helm) pp. 7–16.

Helman, C. G. (1986) ' "Tonic", "fuel" and "food": social and symbolic aspects of the long-term use of psychotropic drugs', in J. Gabe and P.

Williams (eds) *Tranquillisers: Social, Psychological and Clinical Perspectives* (London: Tavistock) pp. 199–226.

Henderson, S. (1990) 'Introduction', in S. Henderson (ed.) *Women, HIV, Drugs: Practical issues* (London: ISDD) pp. 8–16.

Henman, A. (1985) 'Cocaine Futures', in. A. Henman, R. Lewis and T. Maylon (eds) *Big Deal: The Politics of the Illicit Drugs Business* (London: Pluto Press).

Hill, G. B. (1972) 'The Expectations of Being Admitted to a Mental Hospital in DHSS Psychiatric Hospitals in England and Wales', in *Patient Statistics from the Mental Health Enquiry, 1970* (London: HMSO).

Hingson, R. (1985) 'Effects of Marijuana Use on Pregnant Women', in J. C. Gampel (ed.) *Social drug use in society: proceedings of marijuana and health research conference* (Washington DC: Council on Marijuana and Health).

Hite, S. (1987) *Women and Love* (London: Viking).

Hoechst (1988) *Annual Report 1987* (Frankfurt: Hoechst).

Hoffman, A. (1987) *Steal This Urine Test* (New York: Viking Penguin).

Holland, J., Ramazanoglu, C. and Scott S. (1990) 'AIDS: From Panic Stations to Power Relations: Sociological Perspectives and Problems', *Sociology*, 24,3, pp. 499–518.

Holmila, M. (1985) 'The Guardian Angel or drinking companion: the spouse's influence on drinking in young families in Helsinki, Tallian and Moscow', paper presented at the Cultural Studies Conference on Drinking and Drinking Problems, Helsinki, 24–28 September.

Holmila, M., Mustonen, H. and Rannik, E. (1990) 'Alcohol use and its control in Finnish and Soviet marriages', *British Journal of Addiction*, 85, pp. 509–20.

Holstein, J. A. (1987) 'Producing Gender Effects on Involuntary Mental Hospitalization', *Social Problems*, 34, 2, pp. 141–55.

Home Office (1990) *Statistics of the Misuse of Drugs: Addicts Notified to the Home Office, United Kingdom, 1989* (London: Home Office).

Home Office (1991) *Statistics of the Misuse of Drugs: Addicts Notified to the Home Office, United Kingdom, 1990* (London: Home Office).

Hser, Y., Anglin M. D. and McGlothlin, W. (1987) 'Sex Differences in Addict Careers. 1 Initiation of use', *American Journal of Drug and Alcohol Abuse*, 13, 1&2, pp. 33-57.

Hunt, G. and Saterlee, S. (1987) 'Darts, Drink and the Pub: The Culture of Female Drinking', *Sociological Review*, 35, 3, pp. 575–601.

Hurst, M. and Zambrana, R. E. (1980) 'The Health Careers of Urban Woman: A Study in East Harlem', *Signs: Journal of Women in Culture and Society*, 5, 3, pp. 12–26.

Huseman, C., Madison, J., Pearson, P. and Leuschen, M. P. (1990) 'Bulimia as a form of self-addiction', *Clinical Trials Journal*, 27, 2, pp. 77–83.

Idanpaan-Heikkila, J., Ghodse, H. and Khan, I. (1987) 'Foreword', in Idanpaan-Heikkila, J., Ghodse, H. and Khan, I. (eds) *Psychoactive Drugs and Health Problems* (Helsinki: The National Board of Health and the Government of Finland) pp. 5–6.

International Committee for Prostitutes' Rights (1987) 'International Committee for Prostitutes' Rights World Charter and World Whores' Congress Statement', in F. Delacoste and P. Alexander (eds) *Sex Work: Writings by Women in the Sex Industry* (London: Virago) pp. 305–21.

ISDD (Institute for the Study of Drug Dependency) (1987) *Surveys and Statistics on Drugtaking in Britain* (London: ISDD).

ISDD (1989a) *The Misuse of Drugs Act Explained* (London: ISDD).

ISDD (1989b) *Tranquillisers* (London: ISDD).

ISDD (1990) *Drugs, Pregnancy and Childcare* (London: ISDD).

Jackson, J. K. (1962) 'Alcoholism and the Family', in D. Pittman and C. Synder (eds) *Culture, and Drinking Patterns* (New York: John Wiley and Sons) pp. 472–92.

Jackson, M. (1984) 'Sexology and the universalization of male sexuality (from Ellis to Kinsey, and Masters and Johnson)', in L. Coveney, M. Jackson, S. Jeffreys, S. Kaye and P. Mahoney *The Sexuality Papers: Male Sexuality and the Social Control of Women* (London: Hutchinson) pp. 69–84.

Jacobson, B. (1981) *The Ladykillers: Why Smoking is a Feminist Issue* (London: Pluto Press).

Jacobson, B. (1985) 'Tobacco and the third world: a growing "epidemic"', *World View 1985 – An Economic and Political Yearbook* (London: Pluto Press).

Jacobson, B. (1986) *Beating the Ladykillers: Women and Smoking* (London: Pluto Press).

James, B. (1987) 'Women and AIDS: the same old story', *Radical Community Medicine*, Autumn, pp. 4–9.

Jamieson, A., Glarz, A. and S. MacGregor (1984) *Dealing with Drug Misuse*, London, Tavistock.

Jeffries, S. (1983) 'Heroin Addiction: Beyond the Stereotype', *Spare Rib*, 132, pp. 6–8.

Jeger, L. (1965) 'The Social Implications', in C. M. Fletcher, H. Cole, L. Jeger and C. Wood, *Common Sense about Smoking* (Harmondsworth: Penguin) pp. 71–98.

Jellinek, E. M. (1952) 'Phases of Alcohol Addiction', *Quarterly Journal of Studies on Alcohol*, 7, pp. 673–84.

Jellinek, E. M. (1960) *The Disease Concept of Alcoholism* (New Haven: College and University Press in Association with Hillhouse Press, New Brunswick, New Jersey).

Jenkins Gaines, J. (1976) 'Alcohol and the Black Woman', in F. D. Harper (ed.) *Alcohol Abuse and Black America* (Alexandria: Virginia Douglas Publications).

Jessup, M. and Green, J. R. (1987) 'Treatment of the Pregnant Alcohol-dependent Woman', *Journal of Psychoactive Drugs*, 19, 2, pp. 193–203.

Johnson, M. and Auerbach, A. H. (1984) 'Women and Psychotherapy Research', in L. E. Walker (ed.) *Women and Mental Health Policy* (Beverly Hills: Sage Publications) pp. 59–78.

Johnston, L. D., O'Malley, P. and Bachman, J. (1987) 'Psychotherapeutic,

Licit and Illicit Use of Drugs among Adolescents: An Epidemiological Perspective', *Journal of Adolescent Health Care*, 8, pp. 36–51.

Jones, K. L. and Smith, D. W. (1973) 'Recognition of the fetal alcohol syndrome in early infancy', *Lancet*, 2, pp. 999–1001.

Jones, M. C. (1971) 'Personality Antecedents and correlates of drinking patterns in women', *Journal Consultancy Clinical Psychology*, 36, pp. 61–9.

Jopke, T. (1990) 'Pregnancy and Drugs', *Minnesota Medicine*, 73 (4), pp. 29–32.

Journal of Psychoactive Drugs (1987) 'Special Issue on Women', 19, 2, edited by S. Murphy and M. Rosenbaum.

Kail, B. L. and Lukoffif, I. F. (1984a) 'Differentials in the Treatment of Black Female Heroin Addicts', *Drug and Alcohol Dependence*, 13, pp. 55–63.

Kail, B. L. and Lukoffif, I. F. (1984b) 'The Black Female Addict's Career Options: A Typology and Theory', *American Journal of Drugs and Alcohol Abuse*, 10, 1, pp. 39-52.

Kalant, O. J. (1980) 'Sex differences in alcohol and drug problems: some highlights', in O. J. Kalant (ed.) *Alcohol and Drug Problems in Women* (London: Plenum Press).

Kaufman Kantor, G. and Straus, M. (1987) 'The "Drunken Bum" Theory of Wife Beating', *Social Problems*, 34, 1, pp. 213–30.

Kearney, P. (1987) 'Preparing for Birth', *Druglink*, 12, pp. 4, 9.

Kelly (1983) 'The Goddess is Fat', in L. Schoenfielder and B. Wieser (eds) *Shadow on a Tightrope* (Iowa City: Aunt Lute Book Company) pp. 15–21.

Kent, R. (1990) *Say when: Everything a woman needs to know about drinking problems* (London: Sheldon Press).

Kerns, L. L. (1986) 'Treatment of Mental Disorders during Pregnancy: A Review of Psychotropic Drug Risks and Benefits', *Journal of Nervous and Mental Diseases*, 174, 11, pp. 652–9.

Kessel, N. and Walton, H. (1965) *Alcoholism* (Harmondsworth: Penguin).

Khabbaz, R., Darrow, W., Hartley, T., Witte, J., Cohen, J. French, J., Gill, P., Potterat, J., Sikes, K. Reich, R., Kaplan, J. and Lairmore, M. (1990) 'Seroprevalence and Risk Factors for HTLV-I/II Infection Among Female Prostitutes in the United States', *Journal of the American Medical Association* 263, pp. 60–4.

Kinsey, B. A. (1966) *The Female Alcoholic: A Social Psychological Study* (Springfield, Illinois: Thomas).

Kinsey, B. A. (1968) 'Psychological factors in alcoholic women from a hospital sample', *American Journal of Psychiatry*, 124, pp. 1463–8.

Kirkpatrick, J. (1977) *Turnabout: Help for a new life* (Seattle: Madrona Publishers).

Klein, V. (1965) *Britain's Married Women Workers* (London: Routledge & Kegan Paul).

Kline, J. Stein, Z. and Hutzler, M. (1982) 'Cigarettes, Alcohol and Marijuana: Varying Associations with Birthweight', *International Journal of Epidemiology*, 16, 1, pp. 44–51.

Knupfer, G. (1982) 'Problems associated with drunkenness in women: some research issues', in NIAAA *Alcohol and Health Monograph 4: Special Population Issues* (Rockville, Maryland: NIAAA).

Kohn, M. (1987) *Narcomania: On Heroin* (London: Faber & Faber).

Koskowski, W. (1955) *The Habit of Smoking Tobacco* (London: Staples Press).

Kowalski, J. (1984) 'Fat Liberation . . . Some Facts', in H. Kanter, S. Lefanu, S. Shah and C. Spedding (eds) *Sweeping Statements: Writings from the Women's Liberation Movement 1981–83* (London: Women's Press).

Kramarae, C. and Treichler, P. A. (1985) *A Feminist Dictionary* (London: Pandora).

Laban, K. M., Bell, F. M. Vernon, D. and Purcell, E. (1981) 'Women in the Military', *Focus on Women: Journal on Addictions and Health*, 2, 1, pp. 14–19.

Lacey, R. (1984) 'Prescriptions – What Price Official Secrecy?', *Open Mind*, 9, p. 13.

Lader, M. H. (1978) 'Benzodiazepines: the opium of the masses?', *Neuroscience*, 3, 2, pp. 159–65.

Lader, M. (1981) 'Introduction', in C. Haddon (ed.) *Women and Tranquillisers* (London: Sheldon Press) pp. 1–3.

Lader, M. (1983) 'Dependence on Benzodiazepines', *Journal of Clinical Psychiatry*, 44, 4, pp. 121–7.

Lancet (1978) vol 12, p. 946.

Laurance, J. (1987) 'The Happy Addict', *New Society*, 24 April, 80, 1269, pp. 9–10.

Lauy, G. (1987) 'Nutmeg Intoxication in Pregnancy: A Case Report', *Journal of Reproductive Medicine*, 32, 1, pp. 63–4.

Lawrence, M. (ed.) (1987a) *Fed Up and Hungry: Women, Oppression and Food* (London: Women's Press).

Lawrence, M. (1987b) 'Introduction', in Lawrence, M. (ed.) *Fed Up and Hungry: Women, Oppression and Food* (London: Women's Press) pp. 8–14.

Lees, S. (1986) 'Sex, Race and Culture: Feminism and the Limits of Cultural Pluralism', *Feminist Review*, 22, pp. 92–101.

Leonard, D. and Speakman, M. A. (1986) 'Women in the Family: Companions or Caretakers?', in V. Beechey and E. Whitelegg (eds) *Women in Britain Today* (Milton Keynes: Open University Press) pp. 8–76.

Lewin, E. (1985) 'By Design: Reproductive Strategies and the Meaning of Motherhood', in H. Homans (ed.) *The Sexual Politics of Reproduction* (Aldershot: Gower) pp. 123–38.

Lewis, R. (1985) 'Serious business – the global heroin economy', in A. Henman, R. Lewis and T. Maylon (eds) *Big Deal: The politics of the illicit drugs business* (London: Pluto Press) pp. 5–49.

Lewitt, E. M. (1989) 'US Tobacco Taxes: behavioural effects and policy implications', *British Journal of Addiction*, 84, 10, pp. 1212–34.

Lindbeck, V. L. (1972) 'The Woman Alcoholic: A Review of Literature', *International Journal of the Addictions*, 7, pp. 567–80.

Lipshitz, S. (1978) 'Women and Psychiatry', in J. Chetwynd and O. Hartnett (eds) *The Sex Role System* (London: Routledge & Kegan Paul) pp. 93–108.

Lisansky, E. (1957) 'Alcoholism in women: social psychological concomitants I. Social History data', *Quarterly Journal of Studies on Alcoholism*, 18, pp. 588–623.

Lisansky Gomberg, E. (1982) 'Historical and Political Perspective: Women and Drug Use', *Journal of Social Issues*, 38, 2, pp. 9–23.

Lisansky Gomberg, E. and Gomberg, J. (1984) Antecedents of Alcohol Problems in Women', in S. C. Wilsnak and L. Beckman (eds) *Alcohol Problems in Women: Antecedents, Consequences and Interventions* (New York: Guilford Press) pp. 233–59.

Litman, G. (1978) 'Clinical aspects of sex role stereotyping', in J. Chetwynd and O. Hartnett (eds) *The Sex Role System* (London, Routledge & Kegan Paul).

Litman, G. (1986) 'Women and alcohol problems: finding the next questions', *British Journal of Addiction*, 81, pp. 601–4.

Litt, I. F. (1981) 'Substance Abuse among Adolescent Females', *Focus on Women: Journal of Addiction and Health*, 2, 2, pp. 61–7.

Little, R. and Ervin, C. H. (1984) 'Alcohol Use and Reproduction', in S. C. Wilsnack and L. Beckman (eds) *Alcohol Problems in Women: Antecedents, Consequences and Intervention* (New York: Guilford Press) pp. 155–88.

Local Authority Associations' Officer Working Group on AIDS (1989) *HIV Infection: Women and Children* (London: Association of Metropolitan Authorities).

Loudon, J. B. (1987) 'Psychotropic Drugs', *British Medical Journal*, 294, pp. 167–9.

Macdonald, S. (1987) 'Drawing the Lines–Gender, Peace and War: An Introduction', in S. Macdonald, P. Holden and S. Ardener (eds) *Images of Women in Peace and War* (London: Macmillan) pp. 1–26.

MacGregor, S. (1986) 'Services for Drug Misusers', paper commissioned by the Economic and Social Research Council Drug Addiction Initiative, London.

MacGregor, S. and Ettorre, B. (1987) 'From treatment to rehabilitation – aspects of the evolution of British policy on care of drug-takers', in. N. Dorn and N. South (eds) *Land Fit for Heroin?* (London: Macmillan) pp. 125–45.

MacKeith, N. (compiler) (1976) *Women's Health Handbook: A Self-Help Guide* (London: Expression Printers).

MacLennan, A. (ed.) (1976) *Women: Their Use of Alcohol and Other Legal Drugs: A Provisional Consultation – 1976* (Toronto: Addiction Research Foundation).

Madden, J. S. (1979) *A Guide to Alcohol and Drug Dependence* (Bristol: John Wright & Sons Limited).

Madl, R. (1981) 'Myths and Stereotypes of the Sexual Minority Women' in A. J. Schecter (ed.) *Drug Dependence and Alcoholism, Volume 1 Biomedical Issues* (New York: Plenum Press) 903–8.

Mahmoud, F. A., deZalduondo, B.O. and Zewdie, D. (1990) 'Women and AIDS in Africa', *AIDS and Society: International Research and Policy Bulletin*, 1, 2, p. 5.

Mandel, L., Schulman, J. and R. Monteiro (1979) 'A Feminist Approach for the Treatment of Drug-Abusing women in a Coed Therapeutic Community', *International Journal of the Addictions*, 14, 5, pp. 589–97.

Markandya, A. and Pearce, D. W. (1989) 'The Social Costs of Tobacco Smoking', *British Journal of Addiction*, 84, 10, pp. 1139–50.

Marks, J. (1985) *The Benzodiazepines: Use, Overuse, Misuse, Abuse*, 2nd edn (Lancaster: MTP Press Ltd).

Marsh, J. (1981) 'Women Helping Women: The Evaluation of an all Female Methadone Maintenance Programme in Detroit', in A. J. Schecter (ed.) *Drug Dependence and Alcoholism, Volume 1: Biomedical Issues* (New York: Plenum Press) pp. 893–9.

Marsh, J. (1982) 'Public Issues and Private Problems: Women and Drug Use', *Journal of Social Issues*, 38, 2, p. 153–65.

Masini, E. (1981) 'Women as capturers of social change', *Women's Studies International Quarterly*, 4, 1, pp. 95–100.

Mauge, C. E. (1981) 'Criminality and Heroin Use Among Urban Minority Women', *Focus on Women: Journal of Addictions and Health*, 2, 4, pp. 223–39.

Mayer, V. F. (1983) 'The Fat Illusion', in L. Schoenfielder and B. Wieser (eds) *Shadow on a Tightrope* (Iowa City: Aunt Lute Book Company) pp. 3–14.

Maylon, T. (1985) 'Love Seeds and Cash Crops – The Cannabis Commodity Market', in A. Henman, R. Lewis and T. Maylon (eds) *Big Deal: The politics of the illicit drugs business*, (London: Pluto Press) pp. 63–107.

Maynard, A. (1985) 'The Role of Economic Measures in Preventing Drinking Problems', in N. Heather, I. Robertson and P. Davies (eds) *The Misuse of Alcohol* (London: Croom Helm) pp. 232–42.

McCarthy, B. R. and Hirschel, J. D. (1984) 'Race, Sex and Drug Abuse in the New South', *Journal of Drug Issues*, Summer, pp. 579–92.

McConville, B. (1983) *Women under the Influence: Alcohol and Its Impact* (London: Virago).

McNeely, D. A. (1991) *Animus Aeternus: Exploring the Inner Masculine* (Toronto: Inner City Books).

Meis, M. (1983) 'Towards a methodology for feminist research', in G. Bowles and R. Duelli-Klein (eds) *Theories of Women's Studies* (London: Routledge & Kegan Paul) pp. 117–39.

Meis, M. (1986) *Patriarchy and Accumulation on a World Scale: Women in the International Division of Labour* (London: Zed Press Ltd).

Melville, J. (1984) *The Tranquilliser Trap and how to get out of it* (London: Fontana Paperbacks).

Metherell, N. (undated) 'Doubly Dependent: Some Observations on the Rehabilitation of Women Addicts' (mimeo).

Miller, C. E. (1981) 'Counselling Lesbian Women', in A. J. Schecter (ed.) *Drug Dependence and Alcoholism Volume 1: Biomedical Issues* (New York: Plenum Press) pp. 881–6.

Miller, J. B. (1978) *Towards a New Psychology of Women* (Harmondsworth: Penguin).

Miner, M. and Gurta A. (1987) 'Heroin Use in the Lives of Women Prisoners in Australia', *Australia and New Zealand Journal of Criminology* (March), pp. 3–15.

Ministry of Health (1944) *A National Health Service* (London: HMSO, Cmd 6502).

Mitchell, J. (1987) ' "Going for the Burn" and "Pumping Iron": What's Healthy about the Current Fitness Boom?', in M. Lawrence (ed.) *Fed Up and Hungry: Women, Oppression and Food* (London: Women's Press) pp. 156–74.

Moglen, H. (1983) 'Power and Empowerment', *Women's Studies International Forum*, 6, 2, pp. 131–4.

Mondanaro, J. (1989) *Chemically Dependent Women: Assessment and Treatment* (Lexington, Mass: Lexington Books).

Montross, L. and Montross, L. S. (1923) *Town and Gown* (New York: George H. Doran).

Moore, B. Jr. (1966) *Social Origins of Dictatorship and Democracy* (Harmondsworth: Penguin).

Morel, C. (1981) 'Weaving a Feminist Social Work Practice: The Experiences of a Women Focus', *Focus on Women: Journal of Addictions and Health*, 2, 1, pp. 38–47.

Morgan, M. and Pratt, O. E. (1982) 'Sex, alcohol and the developing foetus', *British Medical Bulletin*, 38, pp. 43–52.

Morgan, M. Y. and Sherlock, S. (1977) 'Sex-related differences among 100 patients with alcoholic liver disease', *British Medical Journal*, i, pp. 939–41.

Morgan, P. (1981) 'Alcohol, Disinhibition: A conceptual analysis', paper presented at the conference on Alcohol and Disinhibition, sponsored by the Social Research Group, University of California, Berkeley (February).

Morgan, P. (1987) 'Women and Alcohol: The Disinhibition Rhetoric in an Analysis of Domination', *Journal of Psychoactive Substances* 19, 2, pp. 129–33.

Morgan, R. (1970) *Sisterhood is Powerful* (New York: Vintage Books).

Mostow, E. and Newberry, P. (1975) 'Work Role and Depression in Women: A Comparison of Workers and Housewives in Treatment', *American Journal of Orthopsychiatry*, 45, pp. 538–48.

Mulford, H. A. (1977) 'Women and Men Problem Drinkers', *Quarterly Journal of Studies on Alcoholism*, 38, pp. 1624–39.

Murcott, A. (1983) 'Women's place: Cookbooks' images of technique and technology in the British kitchen', *Women's Studies International Forum*, 6, 1, pp. 33–9.

Murphy, S. and Rosenbaum, M. (1987) 'Editors' Introduction', *Journal of Psychoactive Drugs*, 19, 2, pp. 125–8.

Nairne, K. and Smith, G. (1984) *Dealing with Depression* (London: Women's Press).

National Institute on Alcohol Abuse and Alcoholism (NIAAA) (1980) *Alcoholism and Alcohol Abuse among Women: Research Issues* (Rockville, Maryland: NIAAA).

National Institute on Alcohol Abuse and Alcoholism (NIAAA) (1983) *Advances in Alcoholism Treatment Services for Women* (Rockville, Maryland: NIAAA).

New Internationalist (1988) 'Special October Issue on the Politics of Greed and the Path Beyond', no. 188.

Noble, K. (1987) 'Self-Help Groups: The Agony and the Ecstacy', in M. Lawrence (ed.) *Fed Up and Hungry: Women, Oppression and Food* (London: Women's Press) pp. 115–35.

Nolan, G. and Day, C. (1988) *Alcohol and the Black Communities: Providing an Anti-Racist Service* (London: DAWN).

Norwood, R. (1986) *Women who love too much* (New York: Pocket Books).

Nurco, D. Wegner, N. and Stephensen P. (1982) 'Female Narcotic Addicts: Changing Profiles', *Focus on Women: Journal of Addiction and Health*, 3, 2, pp. 62–105.

Oakley, A. (1981) *Subject Women* (London,: Fontana Paperbacks).

Oakley, A. (1984) *The Captured Womb* (Oxford: Basil Blackwell).

O'Donohue, N. and Richardson, S. (1984) *Pure Murder: A Book about Drug Use* (Dublin: Women's Community Press).

OHE (Office of Health Economics) (1982) 'Medicines and the Quality of Life', *OHE Briefing*, no. 19.

OHE (Office of Health Economics) (1984) *Compendium of Health Statistics*, 5th edn (London: OHE).

Orbach, S. (1978) *Fat is a Feminist Issue* (London: Hamlyn Publications).

Orbach, S (1986) *Hunger Strike* (London: Faber & Faber).

Orbach, S. (1987) 'Foreword', in M. Lawrence (ed.) *Fed Up and Hungry: Women, Oppression and Food* (London: Women's Press) pp. 3–7.

Orford, J. and Edwards, G. (1977) *Alcoholism: A Comparison of Treatment and Advice, with a Study of the Influence of Marriage* (Oxford: Oxford University press).

Osman, S. (1983) 'A to Z of Feminism', *Spare Rib*, November, pp. 27–30.

O'Sullivan, S. (1987) 'Addicting Forces', in S. O'Sullivan (ed.) *Women's Health: A Spare Rib Reader* (London: Pandora) p. 318.

Otto, S. (1981) 'Women, Alcohol and Social Control', in B. Hunter and G. W. Williams (eds) *Controlling Women: The normal and the deviant* (London: Croom Helm) pp. 154–67.

Padian, N. S. (1988)'Prostitute Women and AIDS', *AIDS*, 2, pp. 413–19.

Pancoast, D. L., Parker, P. and Froland, C. (eds) (1983) *Rediscovering Self-Help: Its Role in Social Care* (Beverly Hills, California: Sage Publications).

Parker, F. B. (1972) 'Sex role adjustment in women alcoholics', *Quarterly Journal of Studies on Alcoholism*, 33, pp. 647–57.

Parker, N. (ed.) (1987) *Pharmaceutical Company League Tables* (Richmond Surrey: PJB Publications Ltd).

Parmar, P. (1982) 'Gender, Race and Class: Asian Women in Resistance', in Centre for Contempory Cultural Studies *The Empire Strikes Back: Race and Racism in 70's Britain* (London: Hutchinson) pp. 236—75.

Payne, C. W.(1973) 'Consciousness Raising: A Dead End?', in Anne Koedt, Ellen Levine and Anita Rapone (eds) *Radical Feminism* (New York: Quadrangle Books) pp. 282–4.

Peckham Black Women's Group and The Alcohol Counselling Service (1985) *Black Women and Alcohol* (London: Peckham Black Women's Group and The Alcohol Counselling Service).

Pekurinen, M. (1989) 'The Demand for Tobacco Products in Finland', *British Journal of Addiction*, 84, 10, pp. 1183–92.

Peluso, E. and Peluso, L. S. (1988) *Women and Drugs: Getting Hooked and Getting Clean* (Minneapolis: CompCare Publishers).

Pemberton, D. A. (1967) 'A comparison of the outcome of treatment in female and male alcoholics', *British Journal of Psychiatry*, 113, pp. 367–73.

Penfold, P. S. and Walker, G. A. (1984) *Women and the Psychiatric Paradox* (Milton Keynes: The Open University Press).

Perry, L. (1979) *Women and drug use: An unfeminine dependency* (London: Institute for the Study of Drug Dependency).

Perry, L. (1987) 'Fit to be Parents', *Druglink*, 2, pp. 1, 6.

Petursson, H. and Lader, M. H. (1986) 'Benzodiazepine dependence', in J. Gabe and P. Williams (eds) *Tranquillisers: Social, Psychological and Clinical Perspectives* (London: Tavistock) pp. 44–59.

Philo, R. O., Murdoch, D., Lapp, J. and Mariner, J. (1986) 'Psychotrope and Alcohol Use by Women: one or two populations?', *Journal of Clinical Psychology*, 42, 6, pp. 991–9.

Plant, M. (1981) 'What Aetiologies?', in G. Edwards and C. Busch (eds) *Drug Problems in Britain: A Review of Ten years* (London: Academic Press) pp. 245–80.

Plant, M. (1990) 'Sex Work, Alcohol, Drugs and AIDS', in M. Plant (ed.) *AIDS, Drugs and Prostitution* (London: Routledge) pp. 1–17.

Plant, M. (1985) *Women, Drinking and Pregnancy* (London: Tavistock).

Pollitt, K. (1990) 'Tyranny of the Foetus', *New Statesman and Society* 30 March, pp. 28–30.

Powell, M. (1989) 'The Health Policy Implications of International Trade in Alcohol and Tobacco Products', *British Journal of Addiction*, 84, 10, pp. 1151–62.

Prather, J. and Fidell, L. S. (1975) 'Sex differences in the context and style of medical advertisements', *Social Science and Medicine*, 26: 1183–9.

Priest, J. (1990) *Drugs in Pregnancy and Childbirth* (London: Pandora).

Prusak, B. P. (1974) 'Woman: Seductive Siren and Source of Sin?', in R. R. Ruether (ed.) *Religion and Sexism* (New York: Simon and Schuster) pp. 89–116.

Radical Statistics Health Group (1987) *Facing the Figures* (London: Radical Statistics Health Group).

Ramazanoglu, C. (1989) *Feminism and the Contradictions of Oppression* (London: Routledge).

180   *Bibliography*

Randall, V. (1987) *Women and Politics: An International Perspective* (London: Macmillan Education Ltd).

Rathod, H. and Thomson, I. G. (1971) 'Women Alcoholics', *Quarterly Journal of Studies on Alcoholism*, 32, pp. 45–52.

Raveis, V. and Kandel, D. B. (1987) 'Changes in Drug Behavior from the Middle to the Late Twenties: Initiation, Persistence and Cessation of Use', *American Journal of Public Health*, 77, 5, pp. 607–11.

Ray, L. (1991) 'The political economy of long-term minor tranquilliser use', in J. Gabe (ed.) *Understanding tranquilliser use: the role of the social sciences* (London: Tavistock/Routledge) pp. 136–60.

Raymond, J. (1986) *A Passion for Friends: Towards a Philosophy of Female Affection* (London: Women's Press).

Raynes, N. (1979) 'Factors affecting the prescribing of psychotropic drugs in general practice consultations', *Psychological Medicine*, 9, pp. 671–9.

Raynes, N. (1980) 'A preliminary study of search procedures and patient management techniques in general practice', *Journal of the Royal College of General Practitioners*, 30, 166–72.

Reed, B. G. (1985) 'Drug misuse and dependency in women: the meaning and implications of being considered a special population or minority group', *International Journal of the Addictions*, 20, 1, pp. 13–62.

Reed, B. G. (1987) 'Developing Women-sensitive Drug Dependence Treatment Services: Why so Difficult?', *Journal of Psychoactive Drugs*, 19, 2, pp. 151–64.

RELEASE (1982) *Trouble with Tranquillisers* (London: RELEASE).

Rich, A. (1976) *Of Woman Born: Motherhood as Experience and Institution* (New York: Bantam Books).

Rich, A. (1979) 'Conditions for Work: The Common World of Women', in A. Rich, *On Lies, Secrets and Silence: Selected Prose* (London: Virago) pp. 203–4.

Richardson, A. and Goodman, M. (1983) *Self-Help and Social care: Mutual Aid Organisations in Practice* (London: Policy Studies Institute).

Richardson, D. (1987) *Women and the AIDS Crisis* (London: Pandora).

Richmond, F. (1981) 'Analysis', in *Report from the first DAWN Conference* (London: DAWN) pp. 1–3.

Rieder, I. and Ruppelt, P. (1989) *Matters of Life and Death: Women speak about AIDS* (London: Virago).

Riska, E. and Klaukka, T. (1984) 'Use of Psychotropic drugs in Finland', *Social Science and Medicine*, 19, 9, pp. 983–9.

Robert, J. C. (1952) *The Story of Tobacco in America* (New York: Knopf).

Roberts, D. E. (1990) 'Drug-Addicted Women who have Babies', *Trial*, 26 (4), pp. 56–61.

Roberts, H. (1981) 'Women and their doctors: power and powerless-ness in the research process', in H. Roberts (ed.) *Doing Feminist Research* (London: Routledge & Kegan Paul) pp. 7–29.

Robertson, I. and Heather, N. (1986) *Let's Drink to Your Health* (Leicester: British Psychological Society).

Robinson, D. (1979) *Talking Out of Alcoholism* (London: Croom Helm).

Roemer, R. (1982) *Legislative Action to Combat the World Smoking Epidemic* (Geneva: World Health Organisation).

Room, R. (1980) 'Alcohol as an Instrument of Intimate Domination', paper presented to the Society for the Study of Social Problems Annual Meeting, New York, August.

Room, R. (1983)' Paternalism, Rationality and the Special Status of Alcohol', in M. Grant, M. Plant and A. Williams (eds) *Economics and Alcohol* (London: Croom Helm) pp. 262–6.

Rosaldo, M. Z. (1974) 'Woman, Culture and Society: A Theoretical Overview', in Michelle Zimbalist Rosaldo and Louise Lamphere (eds) *Woman, Culture and Society* (Stanford California: Stanford University Press) pp. 17–42.

Rose, H. (1981) 'Rereading Titmuss: The Sexual Division of Welfare', *Journal of Social Policy*, 10, 4, pp. 477–502.

Rose, H. (1986a) 'Beyond Masculinist Realities: A Feminist Epistemology for the Sciences', in R. Bleier (ed.) *Feminist Approaches to Science* (Oxford: Pergamon Press) pp. 57–76.

Rose, H. (1986b) Women's Work: Women's Knowledge', in J. Mitchell and A. Oakley (eds) *What is Feminism?* (Oxford: Basil Blackwell) pp. 161–83.

Rosenbaum, M. (1981) *Women on Heroin* (New Brunswick, New Jersey: Rutgers University Press).

Rosenbaum, M. and Murphy, S. (1987) 'Not the Picture of Health: Women on Methadone', *Journal of Psychoactive Drugs*, 19, 2, pp. 217–26.

Rosett, H. L. (1980) 'The Effects of Alcohol on the Fetus and Offspring', in O. J. Kalant (ed.) *Alcohol and Drug Problems in Women*' (New York and London: Plenum Press) pp. 595–652.

Rosett, H. L. and Weiner, L. (1980) 'Adverse Effects of Heavy Drinking during Pregnancy: Including the Fetal Alcohol Syndrome', in W. E. Fann, I. Karacan, A. D.Pokorny and R. L. Williams (eds) *Phenomenology and Treatment of Alcoholism* (New York: Spectrum Publications) pp. 139–49.

Rosett, H. L. and Weiner, L. (1984) *Alcohol and the Fetus: A Clinical Perspective* (New York: Oxford University Press).

Roth, L. H. (1987) 'Chemical Dependence in the Health Professions', *Journal of Nurse Midwifery*, 32, 2, pp. 91–7.

Royal College of General Practitioners (1986) *Alcohol – A Balanced View* (London: The Royal College of General Practitioners).

Royal College of Physicians (1962) *Smoking and Health* (London: Pitman).

Royal College of Physicians (1971) *Smoking and Health Now* (London: Pitman).

Royal College of Physicians (1977) *Smoking or Health* (London: Pitman).

Royal College of Physicians (1983) *Health or Smoking* (London: Pitman).

Royal College of Psychiatrists (1986) *Alcohol: Our Favourite Drug* (London and New York: Tavistock).

Royal College of Psychiatrists (1988) 'Benzodiazepines and dependence: a college statement', *Bulletin of the Royal College of Psychiatrists*, 12, pp. 107–13.

Rubin, E. (1975) 'Female Neurosis: A Valid Protest', in D. E. Smith and S. J. David (eds) *Women Look at Psychiatry* Vancouver BC: Press Gang Publishers) pp. 143–8.

Russell, M. A. H. (1974) 'The smoking habit and its classification', *The Practitioner*, 212, pp. 791–800.

Ryle, J. (1987) 'Kinds of Contol', *Times Literary Supplement*, 23–9 October, pp. 1163–4.

Sandmair, M. (1980) *The Invisible alcoholics: Women and Alcohol Abuse in America* (New York: McGraw Hill).

Sargent, M. (1983) 'The Production of Drug Problems: Creating and Controlling consumers', paper presented to a seminar on Exploring the Alcohol and Drug Crime Link, Sydney University, Australia.

Saunders, B. (1985) 'The Case for Controlling alcohol Consumption', in N. Heather, I. Robertson and P. Davies (eds) *The Misuse of Alcohol* (London: Croom Helm).

Savage, W. (1986) *A Savage Enquiry: Who controls childbirth?* (London: Virago).

Schaef, A. and Fassel, D. (1988) *The Addictive Organization* (San Fransisco: Harper & Row).

Schoenfielder, L. and Wieser, B. (1983) *Shadow on a Tightrope: Writings by women on fat oppression* (Iowa City: Aunt Lute Book Company).

Schuckit, M. *et al.* (eds) (1969) 'Alcoholism I: Two types of alcoholism in women', *Archives of General Psychiatry*, 20, pp. 301–6.

Schuman, L. M. (1978) 'Patterns of smoking behavior', in M. E. Jarvik, J. W. Cullen, E. R. Gritz, T. M. Vogt and L. J. West (eds) *Research on Smoking Behavior* (Washington DC: NIDA) pp. 36–65.

Sclare, A. B. (1970) 'The female alcoholic', *British Journal of Addictions*, 65, pp. 99–107.

Seager, J. and Olson A. (1986) *Women in the World: An International Atlas* (London: Pan Books).

Segal, L. (1989) 'Lessons from the Past: Feminism, Sexual Politics and the Challenge of AIDS', in E. Carter and S. Watney (eds) *Taking Liberties* (London: Serpent's Tail) pp. 133–46.

Seltzer, C. C., Friedman, G. D. and Siegelaub, A. B. (1974) 'Smoking and Drug Consumption in White, Black and Oriental Men and Women', *American Journal of Public Health*, 64, 5, pp. 466–73.

Sharpe, S. (1984) *Double Identities: The Lives of Working Mothers* (Harmondsworth: Penguin).

Shaw, S. (1980) 'The causes of increased drinking problems amongst women', in Camberwell Council on Alcoholism, *Women and Alcohol* (London: Tavistock) pp. 1–40.

Shepherd, J., Irish, M., Scully, C. and Leslie, I. (1989) 'Alcohol Consumption among Victims of Violence and among Comparable UK Populations', *British Journal of Addiction*, 84, 9, pp. 1045–51.

Shiell, A. (1991) 'Long-term tranquilliser use: the contribution of health economics', in J. Gabe (ed.) *Understanding Tranquilliser Use: the role of the social sciences* (London: Tavistock/Routledge) pp. 92–111.

Showalter, E. (1985) *The Female Malady: Women, Madness and English Culture 1830–1980* (London: Virago).

Silbert, M. H., Pines, A. M. and Lynch, T. (1982) 'Substance Abuse and Prostitution', *Journal of Psychoactive Drugs*, 14, 3, pp. 193–7.

Singer, M. (1986) 'Toward a Political-Economy of Alcoholism: The Missing Link in the Anthropology of Drinking', *Social Science and Medicine*, 23, 2, pp. 113–30.

Smart, C. (1984) 'Social Policy and Drug Addiction', *British Journal of Addiction*, 79, 1, pp. 31–9.

Smart, C. and Smart, B. (eds) (1978) *Women, Sexuality and Social Control* (London: Routledge & Kegan Paul).

Smith, C. G. and Smith M. T. (1990) 'Substance Abuse and Reproduction', *Seminar Reproductive Endocrinology* 8(1), pp. 55–64.

Smith, D. E. (1975) 'Women and Psychiatry', in D. E. Smith and S. J. David (eds) *Women Look at Psychiatry* (Vancouver, BC: Press Gang Publishers) pp. 1–20.

Snell, W. E, Belk, S. S. and Hawkins, R. C. (1987) 'Alcohol and drug use in stressful times – their influence on the masculine role and sex-related personality attributes', *Sex Roles*, 16, 7/8, pp. 359–73.

Sodergran, E. (1981) *Love and Solitude: Selected Poems 1916–1923*, translated by Stina Katchadourian (San Fransisco: Fjord Press).

Soler, E. G. (1980) 'Women in Crisis: Drug Use and Abuse', *Focus on Women: Journal on Addictions and Health*, 1, 4, pp. 227–41.

Soler, E., Ponsor, L. and J. Abod (1976) 'Women in Treatment: Client Self Report', *Women in Treatment: Issues and Approaches* (Arlington, Virginia: National Drug Abuse Centre for Training and Resource Development) pp. 95–137.

Spallone, P. (1989) *Beyond Conception: The New Politics of Reproduction* (London: Macmillan).

Spallone, P. and Steinberg, D. (1987) 'Introduction', in P. Spallone and D. Steinberg (eds) *Made to Order: The Myth of Reproductive and Genetic Progress* (Oxford: Pergamon) The Athene Series, pp. 13–17.

Spender, D. (1981) 'The gatekeepers: a feminist critique of academic publishing', in H. Roberts (ed.) *Doing Feminist Research* (London: Routledge & Kegan Paul) pp. 186–202.

Spender, D. (1983) 'Introduction', in D. Spender (ed.) *Feminist Theorists* (London: Women's Press) pp. 1–7.

Spender, D. (1985) *For the Record: The making and meaning of feminist knowledge* (London: Women's Press).

Stacey, M. (1988) *The Sociology of Health and Healing* (London: Unwin Hyman).

Stanley, L. (1990) 'Feminist praxis and the academic mode of production', in L. Stanley (ed.) *Feminist Praxis: Research, Theory and Epistemology in Feminist Sociology* (London: Routledge) pp. 3–19.

Stanley, L. and Wise, S. (1983a) *Breaking Out: Feminist Consciousness and Feminist Research* (London: Routledge & Kegan Paul).

Stanley, L. and Wise, S. (1983b) ' "Back into the personal" or: our attempt to construct "feminist research" ', in G. Bowles and R. Duelli Klein (eds)

Theories of Women's Studies (London: Routledge & Kegan Paul) pp. 192–209.

Steinem, G. (1979) 'These are not the Best Years of Your Life', *Ms*, 8, 3, pp. 64–8.

Stephenson, S. (1980) 'Special Issues of Women in Therapy', in J. Dowsling and A. MacLennan (eds) *The Chemically Dependent Woman: Recognition, Referral and Rehabilitation* (Toronto: Addiction Research Foundation) pp. 9–17.

Stepney, R. (1987) *Tobacco* (London: Gloucester Press).

Sterling, S. (1989) 'Benzodiazepines', *SCODA Newsletter*, July–August, pp. 5–7.

Stewart, D. (1984) *Addicted and Free . . . at the Same Time: A Study of Addiction and Fellowship* (Ontario: Empathy Books).

Stewart, T. (1987) *The Heroin Users* (London: Pandora Press).

Stimson, G. V. (1975a) 'The Message of Psychotropic Drug Ads', *Journal of Communications*, 25, 3, pp. 153–60.

Stimson, G. V. (1975b) 'Women in a Doctored World', *New Society*, 32 (656) pp. 265–7.

Stimson, G. V. (1989) 'Syringe exchange programmes for injecting drug users', *AIDS*, 3, pp. 253–60.

Stimson, G. V. Ettorre, E. M., Crosier, A. and Stephens, S. (1991) *Serial Period Prevalence Study of HIV Infection and HIV Related Risk Behaviour among injecting Drug Users* (London: Centre for Research on Drugs and Health Behaviour).

Suffet, F. and Brotman, R. (1976) 'Female Drug Use: Some Observations', *International Journal of the Addictions*, 11, pp. 19–23.

Suurla, L. (1989) *Nainen, Alkoholi, Elämä* (Helsinki: Kirjapaja).

Taylor, D. (1987) 'Current Usage of Benzodiazepines in Britain', in H. Freeman and Y. Rue (eds) *The benzodiazepines in current clinical practice* (London: Royal Society of Medicine Services Ltd) pp. 13–16.

Taylor, P. (1984) *Smoke Ring: The Politics of Tobacco* (London: The Bodley Head).

Thom, B. (1984) 'A process approach to women's use of alcohol services', *British Journal of Addiction*, 79, 4, pp. 377–82.

Thom, B. (1986) 'Sex Differences in Help-seeking for Alcohol Problems – 1. The Barriers to Help-Seeking', *British Journal of Addiction*, 81, 6, pp. 777–88.

Thom, B. (1987) 'Sex Differences in Help-seeking for Alcohol Problems – 2. Entry into Treatment', *British Journal of Addiction*, 82, 9, pp. 989–97.

Thomas, R. M., Plant, M. and Sales, D. I. (1989) 'Risks of AIDS among workers in the "sex industry": some initial results from a Scottish Study', *British Medical Journal*, 299, pp. 148–9.

Thunhurst, C. (1982) *It makes you sick: The politics of the NHS* (London: Pluto Press).

Thurman, C. W. (1983) 'The Structure and Role of the British Alcoholic Drinks Industry', in M. Grant, M. Plant and A. Williams (eds) *Economics and Alcohol* (London: Croom Helm) pp. 249–61.

Townsend, P. and Davidson, N. (1982) *Inequalities in Health: The Black Report* (Harmondsworth: Penguin).

Tucker, B. (1982) 'Social Support and Coping: Applications for the Study of Female Drug Abuse', *Journal of Social Issues*, 38, 2, pp. 117–37.

Turner, B. (1984) *The Body and Society, Explorations in Social Theory* (Oxford: Basil Blackwell).

Turner, B. S. (1987) *Medical Power and Social Knowledge* (London: Sage).

USDHEW (United States Department of Health, Education and Welfare) (1980) *The Health Consequences of Smoking for Women: a Report of the Surgeon General* (Washington, DC: USDHEW).

USDHHS (United States Department of Health and Human Services) (1986) 'Women Intravenous Drug Users and AIDS', *NIDA Notes*, no. 3, pp. 1–2.

USDHHS (United States Department of Health and Human Services) (1988) *The Health Consequences of Smoking: Nicotine Addiction. A Report of the Surgeon General* (Washington, DC: US Government Printing Office).

USDHHS (United States Department of Health and Human Services) (1989) *Smoking Tobacco and Health: A Fact Book* (Washington, DC: US Government Printing Office).

Vaillant, G. E. (1983) *The Natural History of Alcoholism* (London: Harvard University Press).

Valentich, M. (1982) 'Women and Drug Dependence', *Journal of Alcohol and Drug Education*, 28, 1, pp. 12–17.

Vance, C. (1984) 'Pleasure and Danger: Toward a politics of sexuality', in Carole Vance (ed.) *Pleasure and Danger: Exploring Female Sexuality* (London: Routledge & Kegan Paul).

Vanicelli, M. and Nash, L. (1984) 'Effects of Sex bias on women's studies on alcoholism', *Clinical and Experimental Research*, 3, pp. 334–6.

Wagner, S. (1971) *Cigarette Country* (New York: Praeger).

Walker, L. (ed.) (1984) *Women and Mental Health Policy* (London: Sage).

Wallace, R. (ed.) (1989) *Feminism and Sociological Theory* (Newbury Park and London: Sage).

Warburton, D. M. (1978) 'Internal Pollution', *Journal of Biosocial Science*, 10, pp. 309–19.

Waterson, J. and Ettorre, B. (1989) 'Providing services for women with difficulties with alcohol and other drugs: the current UK situation as seen by women practitioners, researchers and policy makers in the field', *Drugs and Alcohol Dependence*, 24, pp. 119–25.

Webster, P. (1984) 'The Forbidden: Eroticism and Taboo', in C. S. Vance (ed.) *Pleasure and Danger: Exploring Female Sexuality* (London: Routledge & Kegan Paul) pp. 385–98.

Weiner, H. D., Wallen, M. C., and Zankowski, G. L. (1990) 'Culture and Social Class as Intervening Variables in Relapse Prevention with Chemically Dependent Women', *Journal of Psychoactive Drugs*, 22, 2, pp. 239–48.

Whitaker, B. (1987) *The Global Connection: The Crisis of Drug Addiction* (London: Johnathan Cape).

White, J. (1984) 'Women and Alcohol', paper presented at the three-day conference, *Left Alive*, November, London, City University.

Whitehead, M. (1987) *The Health Divide: Inequalities in health in the 1980s* (London: Health Education Council).

Wilkinson, J. (1986) *Tobacco: The truth behind the smokescreen* (Harmondsworth: Penguin Books).

Wilkinson, S. (1988) 'The role of reflexivity in feminist psychology', in *Women's Studies International Forum*, 11, 5, pp. 493–502.

Williams, P. (1980) 'Recent Trends in the Prescribing of Psychotropic Drugs', *Health Trends*, 12, pp. 6–7.

Williams, P. and Bellantuono, C. (1991) 'Long-term tranquilliser use: the contribution of epidemiology', in J. Gabe (ed.) *Understanding tranquilliser use: the role of the social sciences* (London: Tavistock/Routledge) pp. 69–91.

Wilsnack, S. C. and Beckman, L. (eds) (1984) *Alcohol Problems in Women: Antecedents, Consequences and Intervention* (New York: The Guilford Press).

Wilson, C. (1976) 'Women and Alcohol', paper presented at USA Air Force in Europe School, London, Camberwell Council.

Wilson, F. P. (ed.) (1961) *Tabacco* (A. Chute) (Oxford: Basil Blackwell).

Wodak, A. (1986) 'AIDS and Intravenous Drug Users', in J. Santamaria (ed.) *Proceedings of a Seminar and Scientific Sessions (St Vincent's Hospital, Melbourne, Department of Community Medicine)* (Melbourne: Maxwell Todd) pp. 179–85.

Woititz, J. G. (1983) *Adult Children of Alcoholics* (Pompano Beach, Florida: Health Communications).

Wolfson D. and Murray, J. (eds) (1987) *Women and Dependency: Women's Personal Accounts of Drug and Alcohol Problems* (London: DAWN).

Women's National Commission (1988) *Stress and Addiction amongst Women* (London: The Cabinet Office).

Wood, H. P. and Duffy, B. D. (1966) 'Psychological Factors in Alcoholic Women', *American Journal of Psychiatry*, 123, pp. 341–5.

Wooley, S. C. and Wooley O. W. (1981) 'Overeating as Substance Abuse', in N. Mellor (ed.) *Advances in Substance Abuse*, vol. 2 (New York: JAI Press) pp. 41–67.

World Drug Market Manual (1986) *Part 1 Europe* (London: IMS World Publications).

World Health Organisation (1979) *Controlling the Smoking Epidemic* (Geneva: WHO).

Yates, G. G. (1975) *What Women Want: The Ideas of the Movement* (London: Harvard University Press).

Youcha, G. (1978) *A Dangerous Pleasure* (New York: Hawthorn Books Inc).

Zola, I. K. (1991) 'Bringing our Bodies and Ourselves Back In: Reflections on a Past, Present and Future "Medical Sociology"', *Journal of Health and Social Behaviour*, 32, 1, pp. 1–16.

Zuckerman, B. S., Amaro, H. and Beardslee, W. (1987) 'Mental Health of Adolescent Mothers: the Implications of Depression and Drug Use', in *Developmental and Behavioural Pediatrics*, 18, 2, pp. 111–16.

Zweben, J. A. (1987) 'Eating Disorders and Substance Abuse', *Journal of Psychoactive Drugs*, 19, 2, pp. 181–92.

Index